"In asserting that 'mental disorders are not equal to madness', Dr. Akita's distinction between psychopathology and madness is clinically, culturally, and spiritually critical. He offers much evidence to support his claim that madness gets lost in the context of Western culture's over-medicalization of psyche. In a world demonstrating increasing madness, this book offers a broader perspective on the dynamic of madness as such and how to differentiate it from psychopathology."

Jerome S. Bernstein, C.G. Jung Institute, Santa Fe, New Mexico, USA

"Iwao Akita's book invites the reader to wander with the author into embracing anew some key issues in psychiatry and depth psychology. His book challenges current psychiatric and psychological paradigms of diagnosis and treatment as too narrow to include the scope and depth of human madness as more than a mental health problem. It is an important book that is right for our time."

Robert D. Romanyshyn, Professor Emeritus of Clinical Psychology, Pacifica Graduate Institute, USA

"This is a beautiful, challenging work. Dr. Akita and his translators have given us an invaluable corrective to the inadequacy and rigidity of contemporary psychological language. The mystery and ubiquity of psyche resists our attempts to contain it in convenient conceptual boxes. Dr. Akita draws us gently back to the questions we professionals most fear, those that remind us of how little we actually know: Why do we suffer? What is the cause of existence? This is not a reflection on the Japanese psyche. It is a gift from the Japanese psyche to psychology."

Sean Fitzpatrick, Executive Director, The Jung Center of Houston, USA

A Japanese Jungian Perspective on Mental Health and Culture

A Japanese Jungian Perspective on Mental Health and Culture: Wandering Madness explores differences between Western and Japanese models of mental health. It argues that while the advent of modern mental health has brought about seminal changes in our understanding of and relationship to those who face its challenges, the cure also seems to be something of the cause, as the classification of mental disorders continues to expand and increasing numbers of people show up to fill them. In this book, psychiatrist and Jungian analyst Iwao Akita presents a new theory of *psycheology* in order to highlight what has been lost in our rush to medicalize the psyche, as well as offer a remedy for restoring balance.

Drawing upon examples from both Japanese and Western cultures, Dr. Akita discusses an alternative perspective to the polarized viewpoint towards which the West tends. He distinguishes the concept of madness from psychopathology and outlines its dynamics through numerous clinical and cultural examples. He describes the underlying dynamics of substance use and personality disorders, makes important links between these conditions, and clarifies how they can develop into madness. With references to familiar stories and myths from Western and Japanese cultures, this book makes an important contribution to our understanding of mental illness and health, while also making us more aware of how these issues are common to the human experience.

This book will be of key interest to academics, researchers, and postgraduate students in the fields of psychoanalysis, Jungian and Post-Jungian studies, and mental health studies. It will also appeal to psychiatrists and other mental health professionals, as well as those with a particular interest in substance use, personality disorders, madness, and cross-cultural comparisons of mental health models.

Iwao Akita, M.D., Ph.D., is a psychiatrist, clinical psychologist, and Jungian analyst. He received his academic degrees from Kōchi Medical School, Japan, and completed training as a Jungian analyst at the C. G. Jung Institute in Zürich. Dr. Akita is a professor in the Department of Clinical Psychology at Kyoto Bunkyo University. He has also been instrumental in the development of analytical psychology in Japan, serving in leadership roles for both the Japan Association of Jungian Psychology (JAJP) and the Association of Jungian Analysts, Japan (AJAJ) over many years. His works now include many publications and several books in Japanese.

Waka Shibata, M.A., co-translated *A Japanese Jungian Perspective on Mental Health and Culture* into English. She is a native Japanese who completed her undergraduate in America and is fluent in English. Since returning to Japan, she has served as the medical director of a medical clinic employing Western medicine, and provided English translation and interpretive services for Japanese businesses. More recently, she completed a master's degree in clinical psychology. Waka is engaged in clinical work while continuing her studies at the doctoral level, where she focuses her research on the Japanese psyche.

Kittredge Stephenson, Ph.D., M.A., co-translated *A Japanese Jungian Perspective on Mental Health and Culture* into English. He is an American who studied the Western tradition (B.A.) and lived abroad in the West (Spain) before engaging with the Eastern traditions. He has studied Chinese and Japanese; lived in Taiwan and Japan; completed a master's in Eastern classics (China, India, and Japan); and published *haiku* and *renku* poetry. He completed his doctorate in clinical psychology with David Rosen, a psychiatrist, Jungian analyst, and *haiku* poet. Kittredge has conducted research on a variety of topics, including the psychology of *haiku*, and works as a psychologist.

Research in Analytical Psychology and Jungian Studies

Series Advisor: Andrew Samuels

Professor of Analytical Psychology, Essex University, UK

The *Research in Analytical Psychology and Jungian Studies* series features research-focused volumes involving qualitative and quantitative research, historical/archival research, theoretical developments, heuristic research, grounded theory, narrative approaches, collaborative research, practitioner-led research, and self-study. The series also includes focused works by clinical practitioners, and provides new research informed explorations of the work of C. G Jung that will appeal to researchers, academics, and scholars alike.

Books in this series:

Jung and Levinas
An Ethics of Mediation
Frances Gray

Symptom, Symbol, and the Other of Language
A Jungian Interpretation of the Linguistic Turn
Bret Alderman

Post-Jungian Psychology and the Short Stories of Ray Bradbury and Kurt Vonnegut
Golden Apples of the Monkey House
Steve Gronert Ellerhoff

Eros and Economy
Jung, Deleuze, Sexual Difference
Barbara Jenkins

Towards a Jungian Theory of the Ego
Karen Evers-Fahey

A Japanese Jungian Perspective on Mental Health and Culture
Wandering Madness
Iwao Akita
Translated by Waka Shibata and Kittredge Stephenson

A Japanese Jungian Perspective on Mental Health and Culture

Wandering Madness

Iwao Akita

Translated by Waka Shibata and Kittredge Stephenson

Routledge
Taylor & Francis Group
LONDON AND NEW YORK

First published 2017
by Routledge

2 Park Square, Milton Park, Abingdon, Oxfordshire OX14 4RN
711 Third Avenue, New York, NY 10017

Routledge is an imprint of the Taylor & Francis Group, an informa business

First issued in paperback 2018

British Library Cataloguing-in-Publication Data
A catalogue record for this book is available from the British Library

Library of Congress Cataloging-in-Publication Data
Names: Akita, Iwao, 1957– author.
Title: A Japanese jungian perspective on mental health and culture : wandering madness / Iwao Akita ; translated by Waka Shibata and Kittredge Stephenson.
Description: Milton Park, Abingdon, Oxon ; New York, NY : Routledge, 2017.
Identifiers: LCCN 2016040778 | ISBN 9781138805699 (hardcover) | ISBN 9781315752105 (electronic)
Subjects: LCSH: Japanese—Mental health. | Mental illness—Japan. | Cultural psychiatry.
Classification: LCC RC339.J3 A35 2017 | DDC 616.8900952—dc23
LC record available at https://lccn.loc.gov/2016040778

ISBN: 978-1-138-80569-9 (hbk)
ISBN: 978-1-138-35376-3 (pbk)

Typeset in Sabon
by Apex CoVantage, LLC

Contents

Foreword

It's a pleasure to write a foreword for such an important work. Dr. Iwao Akita has a similar history as I do, being a psychiatrist and a Jungian analyst. His cases are holistic, and combine his interest in psychiatric medicine as well as analytical psychology. I endorse his approach in using the biopsychosocial model and his addition of a spiritual dimension. Dr. Akita's approach makes sure that finding meaning in madness is an essential aspect of treating our patients. I'm always humbled by William James' philosophy and understanding of how religion and illness intersect. Perhaps Dr. Akita is following the lead of this pioneer by understanding the import of how religion, and its influence on culture, shape our care of patients.

David H. Rosen, M.D.
Eugene, Oregon, U.S.A.

Translators' introduction

The translation of this work is relatively unusual in that it is a collaborative product. At the most basic level, Waka Shibata translated the Japanese text into English, while Kittredge Stephenson refined the language of that translation. However, this description belies the extensive dialogue that was involved to ensure an appropriate balance of accuracy and flow. To speak to the process, then, Waka provided the initial, literal translation of the text. A series of conversations followed with Kittredge to ensure he understood the meaning of the text. An initial polished translation followed that focused on rendering the meaning of Waka's original translation accurately, while making it consistently comprehensible for an English reader with some background in psychology and Japanese culture. Another set of conversations followed to ensure that this level of refinement continued to reflect the original Japanese text accurately. Subsequently, a second polished translation focused on rendering the text into fluid English, with the intention that it read smoothly for native English speakers, as well as capture some of the poetic nuances of Dr. Akita's original work. This polished translation was then reviewed once again by Waka, as well as by native English speakers who varied with respect to professional background and familiarity with psychology and Japanese culture. We would like to thank these individuals for their thoughtful reflections: Sean Fitzpatrick, Bunmi Ogunleye, Ruth Stephenson Strom, and Rodney Waters. At Routledge, Heidi Lowther and Andrew Samuels also contributed valuable feedback. The final translation incorporated these reviews and represents the culmination of these developmental stages.

It is also worth noting that this translation process is itself in parallel with the book's subject. Central to *Wandering Madness*[1] is an appreciation of how Japan and the West each have valuable contributions to make to mental health and our understanding of the human condition. Dr. Akita argues that pooling these different culturally informed insights provides us with an opportunity for a synergetic whole. It is perhaps not surprising that Dr. Akita himself embodies this bridging of understandings, both with respect to Japanese and Western cultures, as well as mental health. As his author description and the book itself make apparent, Dr. Akita's life and experiences are testaments to the insights he shares here. What may be less apparent is that the translation process, and the translators themselves, also manifest this dynamic. The extensive conversations required to accurately translate the work were apposite reflections of this intention to bring Japanese and Western cultures and mental health perspectives into dialogue. This dialogue, in turn, was made possible by Waka and Kittredge's respective explorations and experiences – East and West, cultural and psychological. Thus, the translation of this work has been not only dynamic, but embodied.

Having reviewed the translation process, we would like to discuss a number of points regarding the translation itself. The first is primarily a cultural distinction that is reflected in the respective languages. The Japanese have a distinctive aesthetic and corresponding affinity for images. By way of example, Hayao Kawai was the first Japanese to become a Jungian analyst, and he was eager to share this perspective in Japan. At the same time, he knew the introduction needed to be made with care if it were to be adopted. So he began by introducing sandplay therapy, which provided an opportunity for the Japanese to gain an appreciation for the dynamism of the scenes – images – depicted in this therapeutic mode. As this experiential sense for the psychological power of images was adopted, Dr. Kawai introduced Jungian psychology, which complemented sandplay therapy and provided additional scope and insight through its interpretations of symbolic images. In keeping with Dr. Akita's argument in this text, one might say that the Japanese have an intuitive grasp for the dynamism of symbolic images. In contrast, Western cultures tend to emphasize intellectual comprehension in keeping with Descartes' philosophy.

This cultural difference is reflected in language used to describe the assimilative process. For example, Dr. Akita sometimes uses words that describe an image or the process of viewing something, whereas the rendering in English might use recollection, recognition, or the like. In English, too, one can "see" what someone is saying, but this usage differs from the more direct assimilation of the images themselves that is reflected in Japanese usage. The implication is that the Japanese come into relationship with something more through the process of engaging with images of it, whereas native Western speakers of English place more of an emphasis on cognitive modes of assimilation. In this translation, we have retained language that reflects assimilation through vision and images where possible, but have made use of more cognitively oriented language at times to render a smoother translation or reflect the primary meaning in context.

A second point is to note that the original Japanese text is quite poetic. To read it is to have something of the experience Dr. Akita attributes to the Japanese generally, i.e., that they are able to dance with both conscious and unconscious elements. One example would be his discussion of *The Little*

Prince in Chapter 2. Dr. Akita weaves quotes from *The Little Prince* in with paraphrase and interpretive comments to form a coherent whole. All of this is made more immediate by his decision not to refer to the protagonist of the work in any way other than the first-person pronouns used in the book itself. The resultant effect is to make the reader feel quite close to both the protagonist of the work and to Dr. Akita as he develops his interpretation of it. He is similarly deft in molding his audience into different roles throughout the text. *Wandering Madness* leaves open the possibility, implicitly, that the readers have within themselves the capacity to be mad, to be therapists, and to be clients. In other words, he writes in a manner that invites readers to reflect on the various roles they play in the dynamics he is discussing. Our translation inevitably falls short of capturing such a fluid and poetic style – and indeed, such a perception of life itself.

A third issue that affects the work as a whole is the development of the *Diagnostic and Statistical Manual of Mental Disorders* (DSM). When the original Japanese version of *Wandering Madness* was published in January of 2012, DSM-IV-TR was still current. DSM-5 was released in May of 2013 and did away with the multiaxial assessment system that placed personality disorders on a separate axis than other diagnoses. Dr. Akita discusses this role of personality disorders and their position in the DSM at length in Chapter 4. Given that the discussion of personality disorders runs throughout the text, however, it was decided simply to translate the work as it is, since any attempt to update it so as to reflect the developments of DSM-5 would involve significant changes to the work as a whole.

On a related note, a fourth set of points concerns the terminology associated with clinical practice. As a psychiatrist, a clinical psychologist, and a Jungian analyst, Dr. Akita has an unusually broad perspective on clinical work and the various professions that compose it. Sometimes, the distinctions between the professions are straightforward. In the original Japanese text, Dr. Akita refers most often to psychiatrists/psychiatric medicine, clinicians/clinical psychology, and psychotherapists/psychotherapy. Given his training in multiple clinical disciplines, however, the boundaries between these are not always clear when he shares about his professional experience. In an attempt to capture the inclusive quality with which Dr. Akita discusses clinical work, while also honoring the specificity of the various disciplines, we have chosen to refer to these clinical domains under the general term "mental health" when possible. The terms used for the practitioners themselves have been left more varied. We have generally reserved specific terms like "psychiatric medicine" for those times when Dr. Akita is describing elements specific to that discipline, e.g., the prescribing of medications, or situating it within the history and fields of medicine. Also, while Dr. Akita makes reference to both "clients" and "patients," we have chosen to translate references to individuals seeking mental health treatment consistently as "clients." Finally, there are times when Dr. Akita refers to individuals suffering from mental illnesses in a manner that identifies them with their diagnosis, e.g., a schizophrenic or alcoholic. In keeping with the growing awareness of the potentially stigmatizing nature of such reifying language in English, we have in most cases translated the intended meaning in a manner that also acknowledges the distinction between the individual and his or her diagnosis.

Fifth, it is worth noting that the Japanese language is more contextually driven than English, which involves both practical implications for the translation and reflects a broader cultural dynamic. Practically, pronouns and stated subjects of sentences are often simply implied via context in Japanese, whereas English generally requires them. This issue is further complicated by the necessity in English to acknowledge the gender of those to whom reference is being made. The net result is that, in order to make the translation sufficiently smooth for English readers, we have often had to add specific subjects and referents that are not stated directly in the Japanese. And in an attempt to reflect the gender neutrality of the original work without repeated reference to "him or her," we have often made use of plural forms. Nevertheless, this approach does not fully capture how Dr. Akita balances talking about the individuality of a given client, for example, while situating him or her within the general experience of the human condition.

This issue of context also affects how certain terms have been translated, particularly those referring to evil and the divine. Regarding the former, *mara* can be translated as "evil," "devil," "demon," or "fiend" (from Poe's "The Black Cat," as referenced in Chapter 2). This has been translated primarily as either "evil" or "devil." Our intention was to limit the English words used for a single Japanese term (though variations of "demon" and "fiend" still make occasional appearances), while retaining sufficient specificity to capture differences concerning how *mara* can manifest in a more animated form (devil) or refer to a general force (evil). With respect to the latter, *kami* can be translated as "God," "gods," or "god," depending on the context. Thus, a single term makes reference to the divine as it is represented in the Judeo-Christian tradition, in *Shinto*, and as a more general reference to the divine, respectively. In addition to being marked by context, the particular Japanese alphabet (of three) in which the term is written also clarifies its intended use. In this translation, we have rendered the term in these different forms as best fits the context.

With respect to style and formatting conventions, Dr. Akita makes use of quotation marks extensively in the original Japanese text. As a point of style, for example, he uses direct quotations of his own work, both within the current text and when he cites his previous publications. In English, however, it is common to paraphrase material being referenced in this way. While we retained the direct quotations in certain instances, we often transitioned to paraphrase in order to better capture the flow of the original text for an English-speaking audience. Dr. Akita also uses quotation marks to highlight certain key terms, some of them throughout the text, e.g., "cause of existence," "wound," and "psycheology." In English, however, the convention is to use quotation marks when the term one intends to emphasize first appears, but not subsequently. We handled this differently depending on the term. For the most important terms, such as "cause of existence," "disfigured hero" and "psycheology," we used italics throughout. For other terms where Dr. Akita uses quotation marks, we employed the English-language convention of using quotation marks around only the first use of the term, though this is sometimes repeated for the first instance of the same term in a new section or chapter. Also, we used italics for most Japanese words in the text. Some Japanese terms are sufficiently familiar that they are not typically italicized in English, such as *haiku* or *manga*, but we italicized these for consistency.

Finally, there is the issue of providing Western readers with sufficient cultural context to follow the many references made to Japanese culture, past and present. In rare instances, this additional contextual clarity is added in the text itself and marked with brackets, when the implied meaning is very clear and succinct. The great majority of this information, however, is provided via endnotes. Our purpose is to supply sufficient context to allow readers largely unfamiliar with Japanese culture to read through the text with perhaps only occasional cultural hiccups. At the same time, we have generally refrained from interpretive commentary, trusting Dr. Akita's work to speak for itself, whatever the language.

Kittredge Stephenson
Houston, Texas, U.S.A.

Waka Shibata
Kyoto, Japan

Acknowledgements

Japanese edition

I want to express my warmest thanks to Mr. Toshiyuki Tsuda and Ms. Akemi Watanabe from Sougensha[2] for their support and guidance. Mr. Tsuda was the one who set up this project, and both believed in my potential and worked patiently with me over the course of the book's development. This book would not exist without Mr. Tsuda. He was always encouraging and supportive. He provided me with freedom of thought and expression, which may have seemed rather eccentric at times. He did not hesitate in allowing me to develop my theory. I lack words to describe my appreciation.

I also want to touch upon the cover art.

When I was in Switzerland, I had a dream in which I am looking at a famous Japanese writer, who is writing a novel in a stylish atelier. I had no clue why I had such a dream at the time. Sixteen years later, on November 15, 2011, I visited Mr. Tsutomu Nishioka's studio to discuss the cover art with my editors, Mr. Toshiyuki Tsuda and Ms. Yumiko Miyazaki. (I was meeting Yumiko for the first time, but she contributed greatly to the publication of this book behind the scenes.) As we stepped in, I was confronted with the scene from the dream. That was it! Tsutomu Nishioka and I had several subsequent exchanges through Toshiyuki Tsuda. As someone who appreciates deep questions about the world, I learned a great deal in the course of my communications with Nishioka. When talented individuals get together and work collaboratively, a masterpiece can be produced. Perhaps I should not praise my own book so highly, but when I received the proof for the cover, I felt embraced by the cosmos. I thought, "Finally, this is complete."

Many thanks to Mr. Nishioka, Mr. Tsuda, and Ms. Miyazaki.

I would also like to thank Ms. Natsu Higami and Mr. Hiroshi Sato, who helped me in getting copyright permissions in Japan.

This book was published with the aid of a Kyoto Bunkyo University publishing grant. I want to express my appreciation once again for this wonderful academic research environment.

Acknowledgement of translators

The original Japanese edition of *Wandering Madness* was written in a poetic style with carefully selected language, if I do say so myself. It contains many esoteric Japanese words, rarely used in everyday life. Accordingly, it was a great burden on the translators. Ms. Waka Shibata, who did the initial Japanese-English translation of this book, put enormous energy into clearing this hurdle. The original edition and the translated edition are not absolutely identical as a matter of course, because the nuance of each word is different. Therefore, the original edition and the translated edition of *Wandering Madness* are effectively different works, though Waka's efforts have reduced the gap as much as possible.

It is fortunate that I, as the author of this book, could address Waka's questions directly. I believe this has provided readers of the English edition with a more precise grasp on what the original book attempts to explain.

In addition, I was fortunate to have this initial draft of the English edition developed by Dr. Kittredge Stephenson, who is an outstanding psychologist, as well as a native speaker of English. When the project of translating *Wandering Madness* had just been launched, Kittredge was attending the Graduate School of Kyoto Bunkyo University, where I work and Waka attends. To top it all off, his research topic was *haiku*!

Kittredge is himself an American, but came to Japan to grasp the spirit of this country. The three of us met at such a juncture. Therefore, one cannot hope for a better translation than this. Such an opportunity has been a great blessing for me as the author. I simply thank God for it, as such things are not granted simply through wishing them to be so. Again, I would like to extend great appreciation to Waka Shibata and Kittredge Stephenson.

Copyright permissions

Excerpts from the following authors and titles are published with the following permissions:

Japanese language

Introduction

Nihonteki-kanse, by K. Sasaki, 2010, Tokyo, Japan: Chukoshinsho. Reprinted with permission.

Igyō-ni-sareta-hitotachi [People who were portrayed as divergent] (2nd ed.), by S. Shiomi, 2009, Tokyo, Japan: Kawade Shobo Shinsha. Reprinted with permission.

Chapter 1

Jung shinrigaku nyūmon [Introduction to Jungian psychology], H. Kawai, 1967, Tokyo, Japan: Baifukan. Reprinted with permission.

Chapter 2

Sky-High, T. Takahashi, 2001, Tokyo, Japan: Shueisha. Reprinted with permission.

Chapter 4

Personality-shōgai [Personality disorders], N. Hayashi, 2005, Tokyo, Japan: Shinko Igaku Shuppan. Reprinted with permission.

Chapter 5

Unexploded bomb (Episode 115). *Black Jack* (Vol. 7, pp. 103–127), O. Tezuka, 1987, Tokyo, Japan: Akita shoten. Reprinted with permission.

The second person (Episode 195). *Black Jack* (Vol. 12, pp. 133–153), O. Tezuka, 1988, Tokyo, Japan: Akita shoten. Reprinted with permission.

English language

Introduction

The Letters, by V. van Gogh, 2009, retrieved from http://www.vangoghletters.org. Copyright 2009 by Van Gogh Museum Enterprises B. V. Reprinted with permission.

Chapter 1

The Little Prince, by A. de Saint-Exupéry (T. V. F. Cuffe, Trans.)., 2000, London, England: Penguin Books Ltd. English-language copyright 2000 by Penguin Books Ltd. Reprinted with permission.

Chapter 2

Memories, Dreams, Reflections, by C. G. Jung (A. Jaffe, Ed., R. Winston & C. Winston, Trans.), 1989, New York, NY: Vintage Books. Translation copyright renewed 1991 by Random House LLC. Reprinted with permission.

Takasebune, O. Mori. (M. Brase, Trans.), 2006, Tokyo, Japan: IBC Publishing. Reprinted with permission.

Preface, Japanese edition

When I was working at a mental hospital as a medical intern, I encountered a situation that I never would have expected.

A female client was sitting, leaning against the wall. With her head in her hands, she cried, "I am going mad. I am on the brink of madness!" Her voice was barely audible, forced out with great effort, yet she was screaming with her whole being. Her diagnosis was schizophrenia, disorganized type, which is considered the most severe of mental disorders.

Without this incident, I might never have written this book. Until then, I thought that mad people were those who saw mental health professionals; that when some threshold was reached, they were hospitalized; and that those who were hospitalized were in a state of madness.[3]

However, this hospitalized client with the most severe mental illness screamed, "I am on the brink of madness." What was to account for this?

Were those receiving mental health care not already mad? Was the clinician's role not to cure their illnesses and thus return them to a state of sanity?

Everything I thought I knew fell away in this moment. I was bewildered, having believed that madness resided in mental illness. If those with mental illnesses were not in a state of madness or suffering from madness, and were frightened by the idea of becoming madder, what was this "madness"? Where did it come from? Where did it reside?

– Madness began to wander.

More than 25 years later, I am disposed to submit my own answers to these questions in this book.

> No one sews a patch of unshrunk cloth on an old garment. Otherwise, the new piece will pull away from the old, making the tear worse. And no one pours new wine into old wineskins. Otherwise, the wine will burst the skins, and both the wine and the wineskins will be ruined. No, they pour new wine into new wineskins.
>
> (Mark 2:21–22, New International Version)

In the early days of psychiatric medicine, those engaged in the field must have been quite the pioneering spirits. Pinel liberated the insane from their chains. Kraepelin developed two major psychotic disorder concepts: *dementia praecox* (now known as schizophrenia) and manic-depressive insanity.

Those who had been labeled as mad individuals talking gibberish and were chained, locked up in small cages, or received torturous treatments; were released, acknowledged as sick, and provided with appropriate diagnoses. And the efforts to cure them accelerated. Up to the first half of the 20th century, it was primarily psychotherapy, broadly construed, that developed. From the latter half of the 20th century to the present, new therapeutic drugs have continued to develop. What a blessing these strides have been! While it is regrettable that many have not yet been saved, there are many who have been.

This earliest and most progressive period of psychiatric medicine was a time full of ideas and ambitions. As a development of the Christian nations of Western Europe, however, the field was overly imbued with the Christian ideology. B. A. Morel, for instance, proposed a theory in which the nature of mental disorders was considered a "degeneration," which he understood as a deviation from the norm and traced back to the original sin. He claimed that Adam and Eve's eating the fruit from the tree of the knowledge of good and evil was the root cause.

Although the theory of degeneration was too Christian in its conceptualization, its connections to various fields such as philosophy, criminology, and somatology meant that its understanding of mental disorders was grounded in a broader conceptual context. The theory swept Europe in the 1880s, yet it has been abandoned in little more than a century.

It is no surprise that a theory so heavily influenced by Christian beliefs is unpalatable in our time. Ascribing the nature of mental disorders to the doctrine of original sin could only be palatable to Christian nations. As psychiatric medicine has spread globally, the narrowness of this viewpoint has become apparent. Perhaps this viewpoint should have been preserved in Christian nations, a point I will discuss in more detail in a later chapter.

Thus, the influence of religions and particular ideologies became a huge impediment to the development of standardized criteria that could be applied internationally. This international standard was formed, however, by shedding off layer after layer of these kinds of beliefs, until only a giant skeleton was left. This is the structure that has been presented in *The Diagnostic and Statistical Manual of Mental Disorders* (DSM) by the American Psychiatric Association (APA), a central pillar of contemporary psychiatry, and the "Classification of Mental and Behavioural Disorders" in *The International Statistical Classification of Diseases and Related Health Problems* (ICD) by the World Health Organization (WHO).

Human beings require a skeleton just as much as flesh and blood. Nevertheless, a single rigid structure should not be pursued exclusively. Diversity should exist even at the level of the bones. Of course, the view espoused by the DSM or ICD provides a useful vantage point from a particular framework, but this is only one viewpoint or framework.

As mentioned previously, the development towards internationalization removed the influence of religion and other ideologies. In the process, however, the spiritual elements of these ideologies were also washed away. The religious and ideological aspects were removed intentionally, but this led to the unintentional loss of the spiritual elements as well. As a result, the "spirited" nature of the original psychiatric diagnoses, which carried the imprint of the great forerunners, was lost. In its place, an empty skeleton of a system began to disseminate widely. The present task is to find a way to break through this stagnation. Psychiatric medicine should not remain as it is today. Using the name "psychiatric medicine" is fine since it is a branch of medicine, but its essence should be *psycheology*.[4]

In the practice of modern mental health, clinicians tend to focus too heavily on clients' symptoms, behaviors, or capacities for social adjustment. Moreover, they are obsessively devoted to the removal of symptoms as they are understood in the diagnostic framework. The aspiration to eliminate symptoms has become such an essential part of the relationship between clinicians and clients that it has developed into a fixed, absolute principle. Clinicians now focus on removing the symptoms superficially, as they apply to the diagnostic framework, and have lost their awareness of how the symptoms connect to other elements. But these other elements can serve as a path to the nature of human existence. Such elements include spiritual richness, ugliness, beauty, odiousness, and magnificence – elements that continue to make us reflect on what the core of human existence is all about.

This attitude of symptom elimination has gone too far, such that our present "wineskin" no longer enables us to access the sense of awe at the core of the human psyche.

To share briefly about my background, I trained in psychiatric medicine and Jungian psychology. Since graduating from the C. G. Jung Institute in Zürich in 1996, I have attempted to present novel ideas that might break through the present situation. We need a new wineskin that does not spoil our great forerunners' accomplishments, but rather matures them. In this book, I submit my idea of *psycheology* as a new wineskin, and I discuss "existence" and "madness" as the two axes of a new framework aimed at retrieving the sense of awe, dignity, and mystery in the human experience.

There are four characteristics of *psycheology*. The first is to focus on the *cause of existence*[5] (Akita, 2000). The second is to acknowledge that "objectivity" has no real meaning when dealing with the field of psyche, i.e., objectivity is impossible. The third is to recognize that one's capacity to choose who one really is constitutes the essence of human existence.

However, the question of how to make this choice is a crucial matter. We often elevate ourselves all too easily to the level of God. While those with personhood disorders[6] are particularly prone to the unwitting entanglements surrounding the pursuit of godhood and its resultant disturbance of personhood, such struggles are not peculiar to them. All of us are perilously susceptible to this "illness." I think recognizing this fact is also an important duty of *psycheology*. I will introduce a little prescription for breaking away from this illness in Chapter 4. Therapeutic theory is discussed in the process, so you may note the somewhat different tone of this chapter from the rest of the book.

The fourth characteristic of *psycheology* is that it strives to uncover the nature of madness.

Human beings are subject to wounding. Superficial wounds disappear through the natural healing process. But what if we are existentially wounded? Sometimes we go insane, and sometimes that deep wound itself directs what we must do.

For human beings, when "what we want to do" and "what we must do" begin to intertwine, like the double helix of DNA, we sometimes manifest unprecedented strength – breakdown or breakthrough. Agonizing though it is, such a person must continue to walk in the direction the wound has pointed to in order to avoid falling into madness. When one senses that the breakthrough is possible, the archetype-like power of the *disfigured hero* (Akita, 2001) begins to emerge. The concept of the *disfigured hero* is central to *psycheology*, as well as my theorizing generally, and I describe its most essential points at the end of Chapter 5.

Some additional comments on defining *psycheology* for English readers

It is very difficult to provide a concise definition of *psycheology*. The same issue applies to philosophy, literature, psychology, and psychiatry. A simple definition always risks losing touch with the underlying essence. Inevitably, however, the responsibility lies with the advocate to define his or her terms.

Psychiatry developed as a branch of medicine and became a part of physical medicine. There is no harm in pursuing objectivity in the physical/material domain. In the non-material domain (where the likes of psychology and philosophy reside), however, a single objectivity should not be pursued. This domain should tolerate millions of subjectivities. It should not attempt to extract a single objectivity from a number of subjectivities.

In other words, the pursuit of one subjectivity – God – is all right in the physical world. Making even this statement in such simple terms is far from ideal, but I am using this logic to make the argument for now since this discussion can be very confusing. On the other hand, one truth – God – should not be pursued in the world of psychology or philosophy. A stance that respects multiple or vast numbers of individual truths – gods – is required here.

Two domains (the physical/material and the non-physical/non-material), which are completely different from each other, should not be measured with the same scale. If we call the stance of pursuing the physical/material domain a monotheistic objectivism, *psycheology*, which pursues the non-physical/non-material domain, may be termed a polytheistic subjectivism. It would please me greatly if readers would construct their own *psycheology* as they read this book, while keeping this point in mind.

References

Akita, I. (2000). *Henro-to-sonzai-in* [Pilgrimage and the *cause of existence*]. *Psyche,*[7] *19*, 120–127.

Akita, I. (2001). *Shinriryōhō-to-ningen*: Disfigured hero *Shiron* [Psychotherapy and human beings: Study on the disfigured hero]. In H. Kawai (Ed.), *Kōza shinriryōhō* [Psychotherapy course] (Vol. 6, pp. 111–153). Tokyo, Japan: Iwanami Shoten.

Preface, English edition

I have published a number of articles, but this is my first book. As the publisher of the English-language edition, I would like to express great thanks to Routledge for this wonderful opportunity. The original edition of *Wandering Madness* was published in Japanese in January of 2012. Much to my delight, it has attracted many readers, and was followed by a reprint in 2014. Also, the original edition has been assigned as a textbook or reference book in several universities and graduate schools in Japan, not only in departments of psychology, but also art institutes. As I discuss in the Conclusion, art and madness cannot be separated. I assume this is what led the art institutes to assign the book.

Now, I would like to explain the process of how I came to write this book. After I graduated from Kōchi Medical School in 1985, I continued working at the university hospital as a physician. I was gradually becoming attracted to Jungian psychology under Hayao Kawai's[8] influence, and I left Kōchi Medical School in order to undergo my training analysis with him. This lasted for two and a half years. I then left for the C. G. Jung Institute in Switzerland in 1993, receiving a diploma in analytical psychology in 1996. Returning to Japan, I began teaching at Kyoto Bunkyo University (KBU) in 1997. KBU established the first department of clinical psychology in Japan.[9] Many other universities followed suit, but it is still worth mentioning that this university was the first to establish such a department through the prodding of Dr. Kawai. After establishing the Department of Clinical Psychology, the Graduate School at KBU was formed to offer a master's program, and subsequently a doctoral program. The Graduate School at KBU remains the only graduate school that offers a doctorate in clinical psychology in Japan.[10]

I was fortunate to be hired as a professor at this distinguished university and graduate school. I began teaching students. There was a big problem, though. Anyone engaged in the field of clinical psychology[11] would admit that Hayao Kawai was one of the best teachers. His achievements and influence were extraordinary – everyone benefited from them. As he often said, however, "Two gifts are not given at the same time." In my case, his influence was so strong that I could not help but teach just as he did. It hung very heavily upon me. Those who teach at the university or graduate school level should not be satisfied with mimicking someone else.

Then, in June of 2000, something strange happened. I was organizing paperwork in my office, in the midst of this suffering. Suddenly, the phrase *disfigured hero* popped up in my mind – in English – and intersected with the image of Black Jack, a *manga* character created by Osamu Tezuka. I had no idea what had happened, as the word "disfigured" was beyond my poor English knowledge. I had never used such a difficult word, though I might possibly have come across it once or twice. Nevertheless, this word clung to the word "hero," and the phrase *disfigured hero* struck my soul like a lightning bolt. It was also strange that the phrase *disfigured hero* and the image of Black Jack intersected. I knew of *Black Jack*, yet it was not a *manga* in which I was particularly interested. Still, the image of Black Jack and the phrase *disfigured hero* struck me with equal intensity. I knew immediately that something special had happened to me. Since then, I have been able to talk about clinical psychology through my own words and ideas little by little.

And I finally wrote my first book in 2012, as mentioned above. The contents of Chapter 5 may sound blasphemous to people from a Christian background. However, please do not get the wrong idea. My only point concerns the Bible's lack of a thorough description of Christ after the crucifixion. I am actually a Christian myself. It may be overly bold to compare myself to Jung, who proposed that the Quaternity had replaced the Holy Trinity of traditional Christianity, but I believe I can make a small contribution to the individuation of Christianity by introducing the phrase *disfigured hero* and the image of Black Jack as Christ after the crucifixion. It may sound impious to those who believe that no word in the Bible should be changed, but I am prepared to receive the same onslaught that Jung received from the Church. The assault I might receive, however, would not be as intense given the sizeable initial step Jung took. This is because of the small import of my work compared to Jung's, as well as the historical context. I know I have said this already, but I want to emphasize once again that I mean no disrespect towards Western civilization and Christianity. I am fascinated by the arts in general. Fortunately, Japan has arts with long traditions – *Noh* and *Kyōgen*, each with 650-year histories; *Kabuki*, with a 400-year history; *Bunraku*, with a 350-year history; and *Rakugo*, with a 300-year history[12] – and I have a strong interest and passion for all of them. And yet, if I had to name the greatest artwork of all, it would be Beethoven's masterpieces. I especially love his piano sonatas. They sink deep down into my soul every time I listen to them. They shake me to the core and have a huge impact on me time and again.

As I said, the core of my psychology is *the disfigured* or the *disfigured hero* or the *disfigured self*. There is, however, a problem to consider prior to this topic, which involves addressing the question, "What is madness?" Madness does not mean mental disorders, of course. Yet, we should not ignore the relationship between madness and mental disorders, as they are consciously and unconsciously overlapped. So what is madness, then? For the answer, read on.

Notes

1 Translators' note: The original title in Japanese translates to *Wandering Madness*. While this phrase serves as the subtitle for the English edition, the work will be referenced via its original title within the text.
2 Translators' note: The Japanese publisher of this work.
3 Translators' note: *Kyō-ki. Kyō*: crazy, insane; *ki*: energy, emotion, state of mind, mood. In other words, the feeling of insanity.
4 Translators' note: *Seishin-gaku. Seishin*: psyche; *gaku*: study of (*logos*). See also Translator's introduction.
5 Translators' note: *Sonzai-in. Sonzai*: existence; *in*: cause. In Japanese, this phrase represents a new coinage by the author.
6 Translators' note: In Japanese, what is translated here as "personhood disorders" served as an earlier translation of the English term "personality disorders." The author's preference for this older term is discussed at several points in the work, as well as in additional endnotes, beginning in Chapter 2.
7 Translators' note: This was the journal of the Japanese Jung Club, which was published by *Shinyosha*. The journal is no longer being published.
8 Translators' note: Hayao Kawai (1928–2007) was the first certified Japanese Jungian analyst, who introduced both sandplay therapy and analytical psychology to the Japanese. In the process of doing so, he was deeply influential in both the academic and clinical fields. He was Professor Emeritus at Kyoto University and the International Research Center for Japanese Studies, and was Corporate Advisor to Kyoto Bunkyo University. He was also deeply interested in Japanese culture. He served as Chief of the Cultural Affairs Agency for the Japanese government, and was recognized as a Person of Cultural Merit, a formal Japanese recognition and honor.
9 Translators' note: In the Japanese academic system, departments of psychology have traditionally been housed in other departments, such as education and human resources.

KBU was unique in creating the first undergraduate-level degree in clinical psychology, which introduced a shift from clinical psychology only being offered at the post-graduate level.
10 Translators' note: Since the original publication of this work in Japanese, clinical psychology has continued to expand its reach in Japan, including the opening of additional doctoral programs.
11 Translators' note: Japan has a unique system of licensure for clinical psychologists. Until recently, licensure was managed by a private company. According to this system, an individual must complete an accepted course of study, then pass the licensure exam. Accepted courses of study are either graduate-level training in clinical psychology (M.A. or Ph.D.), or becoming a medical doctor (in Japan, an M.D. may claim to practice in any field of medicine, e.g., a psychiatric residency is not required). Recently, the Japanese government agreed to provide licensure for clinical psychology, which will serve as an alternative and equally valid license to practice as a clinical psychologist. The government licensure

will accept undergraduate-level training in clinical psychology, as well as those mentioned above, with the same requirement that individuals pass the licensure examination. As both licensures will be valid, but the private company's licensure holds to a higher standard of training, it is presently unclear how this will affect the field of clinical psychology in Japan.

12 Translators' note: *Noh* and *Kyōgen* are traditional Japanese performing arts that share a common ancestry and are still often performed together for their complementarity. They originated from a collection of performing folk arts originating in China (eighth century). As they were developed and refined in Japan, *Noh* retained the musical element as part of its highly formalized theater performance, while *Kyōgen* retained the comical elements. *Kyōgen* is often performed as a kind of intermission between acts of a *Noh* play, which is more austere both in form and content.

Kabuki is the traditional dance drama form in Japan. Dating back to the 17th century, its performance troupes were originally women performing both male and female roles. By the late 17th century, the modern-day style was set, in which men perform all roles. The form is known for its distinctive and stylized make-up, costumes, and exaggerated acting.

Bunraku is a traditional form of puppet theater that originated in the late 17th century. The form consists of the narrator (*Dayū*), *shamisen* (three-stringed instrument central to traditional Japanese music) players, and puppet masters. The story and dialogues are narrated by the *Dayū*, accompanied by the musicians. The puppets are roughly one-half life size, with each one manipulated directly on stage by three male performers dressed in black.

Rakugo is a traditional form of comic monologue narrated by a single storyteller. While remaining in the traditional *seiza* sitting position on the floor, and using only a paper fan and small cloth as props, the storyteller weaves a complex and entertaining narrative involving at least two characters, which the storyteller differentiates through variations in pitch, tone, and head position.

Introduction

Madness embraced

The madwoman at the shrine: In the countryside before the introduction of mental health services

Pardon me for starting the Introduction with my private concerns, but I would like to write a little about my childhood. It was the 1950s. I grew up in a country town, a short distance from the center of Kōchi prefecture in Japan. My hometown was only some 10 kilometers away from the central city, Kōchi-city (which used to be a castle town), but in those days I needed to cross a mountain by bus to get there. The castle town was very far, psychologically, and my hometown was isolated from the outside. This created a small, closed world, at least to me as a child.

There were many kinds of people even in such a small world, like a man who suddenly yelled at and beat his wife, and a burly man with glazed, frightening eyes soaked in drink. I've written about this before (Akita, 2000), but there was an inviting shrine near my house. This shrine was an ideal place for kids to play, set amidst a sacred grove, two ponds, a mountain brook, and so forth.

A woman often came to this shrine. She wore ragged, coarse clothes, which seemed long unwashed, and she would totter into the shrine. In the next moment, she would sit down suddenly on the stone stairway and groan, "My head hurts, my head hurts," giving her head painful jabs with her right fist. The kids were sometimes cruel, as they can be, saying, "Go away, you madwoman," or "Stay away – you are dirty." Sometimes the woman would leave, looking sad and in pain; but when the kids went too far – throwing stones, for instance – she would muster what little strength she had to resist them.

Although the other kids pushed her away, I did not dislike the woman for some reason. I sometimes felt a certain sense of belonging and even relief just by looking at her. I wanted to talk to her and bring her some food and medicine, but as a little boy I lacked such courage.

The image of this woman, appearing hungry and wearing grimy clothes, has held fast in my mind. Besides this woman, there were many other kinds of people in my town, such as a crotchety man with a knot between his eyebrows and a woman handicapped by polio.

Nature was abundant around my hometown. There was quite a nice river where I could catch as many fish as I wanted. In the evening, the river became silvered with schools of fish skittering about. The townsfolk lived surrounded by the river, its banks, the clear blue sky and floating clouds, mountains, bamboo, sounds of the temple bell and owls' hoots at night, and the shrine. And those who were more or less odd also lived in this country town as a part of the community, without the names of any diseases being ascribed to them.

This was what the countryside looked like about 40 years ago in Japan. There was no psychiatric medicine in these small towns back then. The hospitals had internal medicine; surgery; ear, nose, and throat; and the like. But they did not have psychiatry – not to mention psychosomatic medicine, which appeared after psychiatry.

This does not mean that mental health services were unavailable back then in Japan. Western mental health already held a place of authority. Designating the starting point of Western mental health is a complex subject, but given that it was around the time when Pinel freed clients from chains, more than 170 years have passed. And more than 70 years have passed since Western mental health was introduced to Japan. My hometown, however, had not yet been touched by its influence.

If the odd people described above were to be categorized according to modern mental health terms, the violent man in my neighborhood might be labeled with a type of personality disorder; the burly man who always drank might be deemed alcohol-dependent; the woman in the shrine might be considered to have schizophrenia; and the crotchety man might be understood to have an obsessive-compulsive personality disorder. Anyway, they were not labeled with such diagnoses, but rather accepted in that town. They lived, embraced by nature, the shrine, and the sound of temple bells – just as they were by the dunghills, outhouses, and the sound of hooves – all enveloping these people in a fine balance.

I did not have any direct trouble from these individuals, but the adults in the community must have had their share of hardship. Even so, the community did not recognize these people as needing to be cured or excluded.

Senichiro Shiomi pointed out an important perspective, which shares the same spirit as my perspective on this issue, in his book, *People Who Were Portrayed as Divergent*.

> The formation of the modern era was accompanied by the discovery of the "divergent."
>
> Soon after the Meiji Restoration, people who had not been considered as odd in the Edo Period, including street performers who walked and

> sang sad songs, those living with animals in the heart of the mountains, or those making bamboo tools, came to be seen as unusual . . . This society considered people who had not been "divergent" at all as "divergent," and was single-minded in its attempts to "normalize"[1] them. What kind of society would do that? When this "normalization" covered almost all parts of the society, the society became obsessed with calling them "divergent," then attempted to deal with them, and finally excluded them. How are these behaviors to be understood?
>
> (2009, pp. 3–4, our translation)

In psychiatry and clinical psychology, an enormous number of people were seen as "divergent" by virtue of the diagnoses they received after the Western mental health system was introduced. Yet, no such concept of divergence existed in places like my hometown, where nature and the cosmos embraced everything as a whole. We tend to see our hometown, wherever it is, through rose-colored glasses. Still, these memories of my hometown are probably not just my imaginings.

No doubt these odd people did face discrimination and suffer. They were also disliked. However, they were not divergent in the manner Mr. Shiomi describes. They were a part of the world. At least, people in that community took such a situation as something that could not be helped. There were the rich and the poor, the landlords and the peasants. Similarly, the sick, the beggars, and the mad were accepted as having their natural place, without any particular consciousness of this decision. Such a feeling was shared implicitly in my community, because all were recognized as part of an unbroken line of births and deaths in such a country town.

Vincent Van Gogh said,

> If we study Japanese art, then we see a man, undoubtedly wise and a philosopher and intelligent, who spends his time – on what? – studying the distance from the earth to the moon? – no; studying Bismarck's politics? – no, he studies a single blade of grass.
>
> But this blade of grass leads him to draw all the plants – then the seasons, the broad features of landscapes, finally animals, and then the human figure. He spends his life like that. . . .
>
> Just think of that; isn't it almost a new religion that these Japanese teach us, who are so simple and live in nature as if they themselves were flowers?
>
> (2009, V. van Gogh to Theo van Gogh, September 23–24, 1888)

I absolutely agree in calling it a true religion. I don't flatter myself to think that the expression of this true religion was present in my hometown, but a slight hint of it could be sensed, I suppose.

Dance of the madwoman

Let's get back to the madwoman at the shrine. This woman staggered about in the shrine sometimes, and it looked as if she were dancing.

Classical *Mai*[2] dance, as seen in *Kabuki* theater, is incomparably elegant. Dancing desperately in a blizzard of cherry blossoms or snowflakes is just beautiful. I call this kind of beauty "mad beauty" or "wounded beauty"[3] (which I plan to discuss in future work). As far as the essence of *Mai* dance is concerned, the dance of the madwoman at the shrine was just as expressive. She danced the beauty of her wound and madness with an ethereal quality. She danced with another world, using every ounce of energy she had left.

Formative *experiences and the existence of the self*

A "formative experience"[4] is "an early experience that greatly influences the formation of one's thought" ("Gen-taiken," 2008, p. 908, our translation). In my case, it was the experience of the madwoman at the shrine, which I now recognize constituted my formative experience as a psychiatrist. I was not aware of it as my formative experience when I first pursued psychiatry, however. Actually, I totally forgot about this woman for a long time. It was about 10 years ago, when I started thinking about madness, that the image of the *Mai* dance of the madwoman at the shrine came back to me in a flash. As I continued to revisit and write about this memory, it became my essential or formative experience.

A formative experience is an early experience that greatly influences one's life. A formative experience tends to be considered something fixed and unchangeable, but actually it is not.

Let's say there's a boy who has been beaten regularly by his father. This frightening experience becomes, as it were, a moving picture or still image projected on the wall of his mind as his formative experience. As this boy grows up and becomes an adult, gathering all kinds of experiences in society, he may come to understand his father's feelings in his own way. Then, the small things that his father did for him may bubble up in his mind and become his new formative experience, which may be more important than the "abusive father" image. On the other hand, he may suddenly remember an even worse image of his father, which might torture him all the more and become his new formative experience.

You can determine what constitutes your formative experience. In your subjective reality, a formative experience is more likely to press itself upon you than your deciding upon it, but a formative experience does not always remain unchangeable. I want to emphasize this point.

A given formative experience might change. Or another formative experience may arise, corresponding to a new level of awareness. People change. For example, a deeper and more appropriate formative experience might surface in parallel with someone's efforts to become more aware and conscious in his or her life.

I would like to expand on this idea that we can determine our own formative experience by referencing the movie *Godzilla: Final Wars* (2004). In the movie, Xiliens of the Planet X come to Earth with a plan to conquer it. Ozaki, the protagonist who is part of a group battling the Xiliens, discovers that he inherited genes from them. He is an Earthman and Xilien hybrid. He loses himself, and feels torn between the Earthmen and Xiliens. After various twists and turns in the plot, he remembers a phrase of Mothra's messenger, and ultimately concludes for himself, "We can determine who we are."

This is very important. We ourselves can determine what to consider our formative experience and our existence. No, we must do so. We must choose one existence out of the many possible ones.

It is also preferable if this existence is not single-layered. This may sound contradictory, but choosing one existence is different from the question of whether that existence is single-layered. Ozaki could maintain higher awareness of his Earthman nature by choosing to be an Earthman despite his not being a pure-blooded one. His choice to live his life in the midst of this irresolvable tension made his existence multi-layered.

As an added note, a previous formative experience and a new formative experience are connected to each other in most cases. In fact, the previous formative experience often manifests its transformation into the new formative experience as a deepening of the previous one. In other cases, however, it transforms into something completely different. In such cases, the new formative experience plunges a person into crisis because the very foundation is transformed. The cracks or splits caused by this shift can accompany pathological as well as creative experiences.

What I want to emphasize here is that, although a pathological experience and a creative experience can be separated conceptually, they do not exist independently. When a thing is conceptualized, its reality splits from its context. This is a disease of modernity, one that tends to be seen more prominently in the West.

In November of 2009, I invited Ruth Ammann, then president of the International Society for Sandplay Therapy, to Kyoto Bunkyo University, where I work, for a symposium entitled "Sandplay Therapy from the Perspective of the Japanese Psyche." I participated both as a moderator and presenter, and found it to be quite interesting. Ammann said something like, "The

Japanese people put their unconscious into words when they use words." I think this tendency also appears when the Japanese conceptualize things. That is, there is a possibility that when the Japanese develop a concept, they put more of the unconscious into it than Westerners. The Japanese may have a tendency to develop a concept without too much separation from reality.[5]

Ammann is Swiss. She said, "Switzerland is surrounded by mountains and different cultures, while Japan is surrounded by the ocean." Nothing is surprising about this fact, but on second thought, it is also quite interesting. Switzerland is bounded by something high (mountains), while Japan is bounded by something low (the ocean). Switzerland is surrounded by the many (cultures), while Japan is surrounded by the one (the ocean, the deep unconscious). Of course, it is unreasonable to consider Switzerland as representative of the West as a whole; but if we use Switzerland as a point of comparison from the West, such an environment surrounded by something high, in addition to various cultures, probably has a tendency to promote towering conceptualization. No wonder a number of concepts that distinguish one thing from another have arisen throughout the history of Europe, which involved a series of battles against neighboring countries of differing cultures.

Japan is surrounded by the ocean. Is this low boundary easier to cross, then? No, it is quite the contrary. The ocean is far more difficult to extend beyond than high mountains. Though low, the ocean is hard to cross. And this low boundary changes dynamically on occasion. This feature definitely has an impact on the Japanese manner of expression: sometimes peaceful, sometimes unsettled, and occasionally vengeful. (It is just like the tsunami that struck eastern Japan in March of 2011. Such a display of nature's madness serves to express a form of the world's psychopathology.) The ocean is also the deep unconscious. As Ammann said, it is quite right that the Japanese, who have been living with the feeling and awareness of the ocean, tend to include the unconscious in their expressions.

Ammann has a receptive attitude as a Jungian analyst and clinician, so she tries to understand others as much as possible. Therefore, she kindly said, "The Japanese people put their unconscious into words when they use words," but many Westerners consider the Japanese manner of expression to be vague and confusing.

Psycheology that dances with the shadow

As Ammann said, it is true that the Japanese are conscious with the unconscious. In fact, the Japanese do not have a mental attitude inclined towards splitting reality themselves. The Japanese psychology has been changing rapidly since the Meiji Restoration.[6] Through this splitting of reality, the

Japanese have become almost too accustomed to expressing themselves in a manner that is either pathological or creative.

This point must be well recognized. A concept or a word is much more powerful than is generally understood. If you define or say something, it comes to be.

I can say in this way that pathological experiences and creative experiences do not exist separately. In order to acquire this mental attitude, you need to have the right word and image to describe the experience. This was my intention in describing it as "dancing with the shadow" or "dancing with madness."

The origin of the Japanese word *kage* (shadow) is quite different from what is generally perceived nowadays. Kenichi Sasaki wrote beautifully about *kage* as follows:

> Being so accustomed to scientific reasoning, we cannot help but be charmed by the mysterious aura that the word *kage* creates. For one thing, *kage* means shadow and light at the same time. This strange double meaning appears to be derived from its Chinese character. In short, *kage* means shadow and light, as well as the figure of the object . . . *Omo-kage* [face-shadow] is a word based on this third meaning of *kage* . . . It is difficult to deny that *the sensibility of taking light and shadow as identical* was notable in the ancient world. For instance, consider how we perceive the words *hi-kage* [sun-shadow] and *tsuki-kage* [moon-shadow]. *Hi-kage* is an everyday word to indicate a place out of the sun, in contrast to *hi-nata* [place in the sun]. In Chinese characters, *hi-kage* is written as 日陰, while *tsuki-kage*, a poetic diction to indicate the moonlight, is written as 月影.
>
> (2010, pp. 119–120, emphasis added, our translation)

If we come down to the level at which light and shadow are sensed as identical, the phrase "dancing with the shadow" is no longer necessary. However, the sensibility that would take light and shadow as identical is far from the consciousness of modern Japanese people. Perhaps it is because the Japanese have become too familiar with the Western sensibility, which discriminates between light and shadow. Although far from the level of consciousness, this original sensibility is still alive at the depths of the Japanese psyche. In order to revive this sensibility in this modern world, I propose the way of "dancing with the shadow" or "dancing the shadow." I hope that this proposal will raise new questions and awaken this sensibility of the Japanese psyche in the field of clinical psychology in Japan, where the Western attitude of integrating the shadow into the ego has become too familiar.

Sasaki also discussed the differences in Western and Japanese sensibilities by contrasting the Western attitude in appreciating a rose to the Japanese attitude in appreciating cherry blossoms. Western consciousness is a "one-point focus," (p. 254) which has a person fixate on the beauty of the rose. "In contrast to this intellectual sensibility of the West, which concentrates on an object, the Japanese psyche is in its essence sensuous." The Japanese do not stare at cherry blossoms. They "sense them, not as objects, but as the spreading atmosphere that envelops them." He then quoted a poem written by Akiko Yosano: "People walking across Gion into Kiyomizu for cherry blossom viewing under moonlight are all beautiful tonight"[7] (as cited in Sasaki, 2010, our translation). Sasaki said, "[The poem] depicts cherry blossoms pouring their beauty even onto people who do not stare at them directly, making them beautiful and happy. The spreading and enveloping space of beauty has a long tradition" (pp. 253–254).

Speaking of enveloping, I would like to add one more point.

In October of 2011, I invited the internationally acclaimed Japanese drummers, Kodō, to Kyoto Bunkyo University for a performance and discussion. When I first saw them perform about 20 years ago, I was so overwhelmed by the tremendous sound of the drumming that my heart almost skipped a beat. Two decades later, I was surprised to find that it sounded quite differently. The drumming enveloped me; in terms of the sound, it was just as overwhelming as 20 years ago. But to my astonishment, it was enveloping rather than piercing.

All the performers were in perfect order and harmony, starting and ending their numbers with great accuracy. In such an advanced harmony, the tremendous sound was heard simultaneously as no sound at at all – "What stillness: cicada cries sink into rocks" (Bashō, 1702/1979, p. 46, our translation). It is a phenomenon that is only possible in an advanced attunement, as in a vast wilderness.

Another surprise occurred as they were performing a number entitled "*Miyake*," and I was idly wondering about the drum's potential pain in being beaten from both sides: the drum started to dance. Of course, the drum was not actually dancing, but it appeared as if it were; it began to look like it was dancing with joy and excitement. Motofumi Yamaguchi, the principal member of Kodō, told me that air resides inside the drum – and also god (*kami*). I assume the vibrations reached the god inside the drum and the god began to dance, which might make the drum look as though it were dancing. Later, I learned that "*Miyake*" is a number used for a festival[8] on Miyake Island. My sense of it did not seem to be entirely off the mark.

In another number entitled "*Ōdaiko*" ("Big Drum"), one performer wearing nothing but a loincloth beat a huge drum valiantly. It was totally overwhelming, but in contrast to "*Miyake*," the huge drum did not dance. The drum remained firmly grounded. Probably a variety of gods, including a dancing god and a grounded god, reside in each drum, enveloping us with sound.

Roses, cherry blossoms, and Japanese drums.

The consciousness of the West stares at roses and symptoms. The consciousness of Japan does not contain such an attitude. Rather, it envelops and embraces symptoms. I mentioned that nature and the shrine enveloped the odd people in my country town. Now I think that the "normal" people in my country town might also have been enveloped and embraced by the gods residing in the odd people.

Notes

1 Translators' note: In Japanese, the terms "disfigured" and "normalized" are more closely translated as "different form/dysmorphic" and "same form/isomorphic."
2 Translators' note: *Mai* is a traditional Japanese dance, which is characterized by horizontal movements, rather than the more typical vertical orientation.
3 Translators' note: *Kyō-bi* or *shō-bi*, respectively. *Kyō*: madness; *shō*: wound; and *bi*: beauty. Thus, a certain beauty to be found in madness or woundedness. In Japanese, these expressions represent a new coinage by the author.
4 Translators' note: *Gen-taiken*. *Gen*: original, archaic; *taiken*: experience.
5 Translators' note: Reality, as it is understood here, is a reflection of the whole, which consists of both conscious and unconscious factors in human experience.
6 Translators' note: 1868–1912.
7 Translators' note: Gion and Kiyomizu are popular districts in Kyoto for spring cherry blossom viewing.
8 Translators' note: The term for "festival" in Japanese primarily refers to festivals associated with the native Shinto religion. The *kami* are the Shinto deities, thus the author makes a link between the Kodō piece and the *kami*.

References

Akita, I. (2000). *Seishinigaku-jyo: Kyōki-towa-nanika* [Introduction to psychiatric medicine: What is madness?]. In The Department of Clinical Psychology at Kyoto Bunkyo University (Ed.), *The rinshōshinri-gakka* [The department of clinical psychology] (pp. 157–166). Osaka, Japan: Sougensha.

Bashō, M. (1979). *Oku-no-hosomichi* [The narrow road to the interior]. Tokyo, Japan: Iwanami Bunko. (Original work published 1702)

Gen-taiken [Formative experience]. (2008). In I. Shinmura (Ed.), *Kōjien* (6th ed.). Tokyo, Japan: Iwanami Shoten.

Sasaki, K. (2010). *Nihonteki-kansei*. Tokyo, Japan: Chukoshinsho.

Shiomi, S. (2009). *Igyō-ni-sareta-hitotachi* [People who were portrayed as divergent] (2nd ed.). Tokyo, Japan: Kawade Shobo Shinsha.

Society. (1966). In *The Random House dictionary of the English language* (unabridged ed.). New York, NY: Random House.

van Gogh, Vincent (1888, September 23–24). [Letter to Theo van Gogh]. In L. Jansen, H. Luijten, & N. Bakker (Eds.), *The letters* (2009). Retrieved from http://www.vangoghletters.org

Chapter 1

On the question of why

Constellation

The odd people who stood out in my early experience were the madwoman at the shrine (schizophrenia), the drinking man (alcohol dependency), and the violent man (personhood disorder).

After finishing my basic training as an intern at the university hospital, the first place I was sent was a specialized hospital for alcoholism. The clinical work with addicts was quite hard, and my energy was drained every day. Yet, I was absorbed in this field, thinking that drug and alcohol dependency might become my specialty. After a while, I had the opportunity to study at the C. G. Jung Institute in Zürich, Switzerland. After returning home from Switzerland, opportunities to lecture and write about personhood disorders began rolling in, which then absorbed me for some time.

As Agatha Christie (1944) said through one of her characters, "The story begins long before that – years before sometimes . . . And then, when the time comes . . . all of [it] converg[es] towards zero" (pp. 12–13). My journey as a psychiatrist "begins long before that," at least as early as when I received strong impressions from the odd people in my town, such as the drinking man and the violent man. I might have unconsciously formed what "begins long before that" as a question to be asked of life. As it was, my clinical work and research on alcohol dependence and personhood disorders seemed to converge "towards zero." It was downright strange. I cannot take it as just a coincidence, nor do I feel myself simply to be making it up. In retrospect, each instance seems to have been inevitable, though it never felt that way during my journey.

The drinking man and the violent man did have some sort of influence on my life. What I mean by influence here is something that shapes one's destiny, something that moves one subtly yet powerfully in the psychic depths. In Jungian psychology, such a condition that is brought on with this kind of power is called a "constellation," using an analogy from the stars at night.

The cause of existence

As for a mental attitude conducive to the discovery of such constellations, I would suggest one of leaning into the *cause of existence.*

It was when I wrote a paper entitled "Pilgrimage and the *Cause of Existence*" (Akita, 2000) 10 years ago that I used this term for the first time. Drawing on this paper, let me explain what the *cause of existence* is about.

Around the time I was writing this paper, etiology was an important research question for me. Etiology is the cause of a disease, and in psychiatric medicine, the cause is described using terms such as endogenous cause, exogenous cause, or psychogenic cause. Here is how modern Western psychiatry categorizes the cause or formation of mental disorders. First, the cause is determined to be either a physiological or a psychogenic cause. Second, a physiological cause is determined to be either an endogenous cause or an exogenous cause (Figure 1.1). The endogenous type of physiological cause means a cause that is undefined as of yet, but whose biological base is expected to be understood in the future; schizophrenia and bipolar disorder are categorized as endogenous mental disorders. The exogenous type of physiological cause is often referred to simply as the exogenous cause, because the mental disorders with this cause can be explained in terms of physiological pathology: infection, intoxication, degeneration, and external injury are in this category. The subcategories of exogenous causes in psychiatric medicine are organic psychoses, symptomatic psychoses, and mental disorders related to substances such as drugs and alcohol. The term psychogenic cause is used when a mental conflict is the cause of the mental disorder, such as a neurosis.

This taxonomy has as its central axis the distinction between the physiological cause and the psychological cause. There is another taxonomy that places the endogenous cause versus the exogenous cause at the center (Figure 1.2). Both the physiological–psychological cause axis and the endogenous–exogenous cause axis follow the two-category system: body–mind and endogenous–exogenous. The two-category system can provide

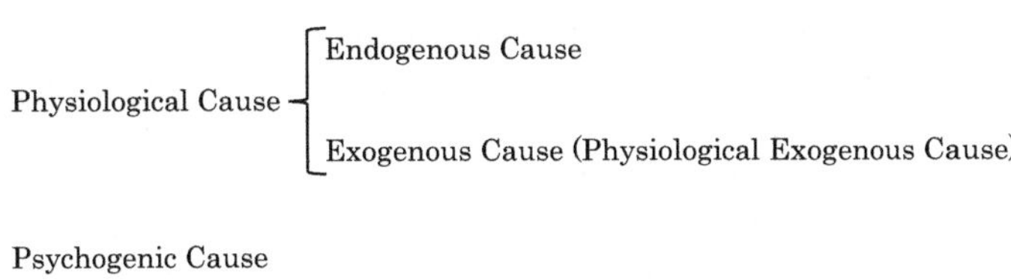

Figure 1.1

- Endogenous Cause
- Exogenous Cause
  - Physiological Exogenous Cause
  - Psychogenic Cause

Figure 1.2

a makeshift scientific explanation, but this dichotomy cannot answer the "why" question, as Kawai pointed out as early as 1967. Kawai said:

> A man[1] lost his fiancée in a traffic accident right before the wedding. He asks, "Why?" "Why did my fiancée die?" A doctor would answer, "It is due to the head injury, and . . . ." This answer is not incorrect. Yet, it will not satisfy him. How come this correct answer does not satisfy him? It is because the answer was given by converting the question of "why" to the question of "how" . . . In other words, natural science has accomplished today's development by shifting from "why" to "how."
>
> (1967, pp. 2–3, our translation)

Unfortunately, the mental stance intent upon answering "why" questions is absent from the etiology of modern psychiatry. Once psychiatric medicine was incorporated into natural science, which had been developing by shifting from "why" to "how," this was inevitable. It is a big issue for psychiatric medicine. What is worse, the issue is so large that even locating the problem is difficult. As the proverb says, "You can't see the forest for the trees." This forest is massive.

Psychiatric medicine, which should hold "why" questions at its center, must not be positioned merely as a branch of natural science. As long as it is positioned as psychiatric *medicine*, however, it can only function as a branch of medicine, which in turn serves as a branch of natural science. Getting out of this dilemma begins with recognizing this fact. Then, psychiatric medicine needs to shed its skin and regenerate towards *psycheology*.

Clients come on a daily basis. Psychiatric medicine is needed, i.e., psychiatric medicine needs to remain a branch of medicine. However, when psychiatric medicine substantially individuates itself as *psycheology* – that is, when psychiatric medicine maintains an attitude that concerns itself with "why" questions – it can soar into *psycheology*, which can transcend the logic of natural science. Such a spirit also needs to extend into other branches of medicine, because "why" questions overflow into all medical branches. Psychiatric medicine as *psycheology* needs to develop itself enough to exist in and support all of the other branches, including internal and emergency medicine. When Western medicine attains this perspective, the forest called psychiatric medicine, which includes even the woods of psychiatric medicine as *psycheology,* can become luxuriant and provide people with true rest.

Although the clinical practice of psychiatry is full of these "why" questions, the mental attitude to support answering them cannot be found in its etiology. The psychogenic cause is ostensibly responsible for addressing "why" questions, but it tends to be handled in the context of "how," so "why" is once again excluded. Should the etiology of the psychogenic cause just grow and expand to the point of addressing "why" questions, then? That is not enough – because mental disorders due to endogenous and exogenous causes also carry "why" questions.

It is these "why" questions that house the attitude of searching for one's *cause of existence*. The conceptual utility of endogenous, exogenous, and psychogenic causes does not need to be questioned. Clinicians, however, must be aware of the *cause of existence* in order to avoid ignoring the "why" questions that lurk and swirl in the abyss, and thus to be of help to those searching for their individuality. When the thirst for the *cause of existence* remains unquenched, some people step into fortune-telling, or even shady cults.

What is the *cause of existence*?

When therapists attempt to attune to their clients' *cause of existence*, it provides a space in which clients can open into their individuality. It is this attitude that is necessary for psychiatric medicine itself to open up.

I have been using the phrase *cause of existence* without any definition so far in the hopes that you might get a sense for it, as this term can only be understood intuitively. Even so, I will add the following tentative explanation.

The intension[2] of "existence" in the term *cause of existence* is "being." No doubt about it. Descartes said, "I think, therefore I am" (1637/1952, p. 51). The "I" who thinks, or the ego, becomes the foundation of cognitive certainty. This has been the foundation for the conventional etiology of Western psychiatric medicine. In contrast, if we posit the *cause of existence* as underpinning a physiological, psychogenic, endogenous, or exogenous cause, the foundation for cognitive certainty becomes, "I am, therefore I am" (Figure 1.3). Furthermore, concepts such as fate, soul, Self, karma, reincarnation, cosmos, the law of causation, God, the devil, the collective unconscious, as well as the problems and tasks of humanity, can all be seen as extensions of this being.

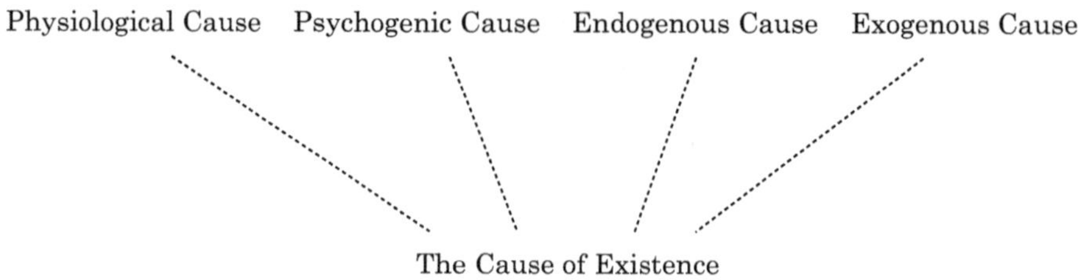

Figure 1.3

Ten years ago, I wrote:

> By the way, if you ask me whether I can conduct psychotherapy with the attitude of attuning myself to the *cause of existence* in my clinical practice, I am not 100% sure. Of course I am trying, but when I reflect on my clinical work in psychiatry, sometimes I see clients while distracted by my own thoughts, such as "Oh, I'm hungry," or "I want to go home and watch the evening game with a glass of beer." If clients saw into my mind, they might get angry.
>
> (2000, p. 124, our translation)

I may have grown a bit since then, because such distractions rarely occur in therapy nowadays. Even if such worldly thoughts show up, I just let them flow around the rim of consciousness as worldly thoughts, rather than getting caught up in them, and I direct my mind straight into the essence that needs to be approached. The worldly thoughts may not have decreased so much as they have become less sticky.

I continued as follows:

> However, when a therapist, who struggles with these worldly, evil, and delusional thoughts, still tries to be attuned in a prayerful fashion, sometimes the *cause of existence* can be seen intuitively in a moment of purity. Guggenbühl-Craig, one of my analysts, told me that there was also a time when he struggled with questions of why he had to live. When he looked at the mountain from the window, he suddenly realized, "Now I see – that's it."[3] I wonder if this is similar to when one glimpses the *cause of existence* intuitively. Then, the internal process begins again, tracing the path of this new "opening."
>
> I wrote, "struggles with these worldly . . . thoughts," but speaking candidly from my own experience, these worldly thoughts seem to be rather necessary sometimes to intuit the *cause of existence*, which enable

> one to survive this life. When we try to reach out towards this "opening" for living, these sloppy thoughts might be essential ingredients.
> (p. 124)

This is also a bit different from how I perceive things now. You may think that I should limit myself to discussing only the most developed or latest ideas that have come to me with more experience. Assuming that the ages and experiences of readers will vary, however, I decided to include my clinical approach to this 10 years ago in the hopes that it may be of some use.

As I mentioned, I suffer less from worldly, evil, or delusional thoughts than before. At the same time, the sense of bringing a prayerful attitude into psychotherapy has decreased as well. No. Rather, I would like to believe that this attitude has been acquired to the point that I don't have to be so aware of this sense of praying anymore. I use the term "believe" because, despite this process taking place within myself, it is too delicate for me to be sure.

I used to be keenly aware of evil influences, so the sense of praying also stood out to me. But the boundary between evil, worldly, obsessive, and delusional thoughts has become more vague with time. This applies to prayer as well. The purity with which prayer is practiced and the ends it is asked to serve differ depending on one's perspective – it is the prayerful intention that is holy.

My present clinical approach is to direct my mind towards the *cause of existence*, while letting everything – including evil, worldly, and prayerful thoughts – float around the extension of the existence. I feel like I am slowly sinking down towards the *cause of existence* in order to catch a glimpse of something ethereal. I protect myself with only a thin layer of psychological cosmetics (*kokoro-gesō*),[4] attempting to descend with a mind as free from worldly thoughts as possible. The degree of freedom is much higher than before, as worldly thoughts have become less sticky. My ability to reach further to the right, left, forward, and backward seems to have increased.

The little prince

Many of you may know *The Little Prince*, a story written by Saint-Exupéry (1943/2000).

The little prince was too pure, innocent, ephemeral, frail, and vulnerable. He was looking for something very important, yet he wandered aimlessly. (It is like being sent out too far and wandering beautifully amidst the melody of Beethoven's "Moonlight Sonata" while the soul seeks for something important but out of sight.) The little prince's situation of having no place to go is almost painful. When existential concerns are touched upon, the little prince – the *cause of existence* – is shaken within us. Then something can be sensed.

Sometimes I sense this in sitting with a client. I attempt to be as open as possible without losing a sense of myself, sitting in front of this other without knowing who the client really is.

After the journey around the planets, the little prince came to Earth and met the pilot who narrates the story. Time passed, and the little prince let a poisonous snake bite his body. His body had become too heavy to travel, so he abandoned it and returned to his planet. This internationally beloved story is no doubt wonderful as it is, yet the little prince being bitten and then dying is still sad. Before I wrote, "Slowly sinking down towards the *cause of existence* in order to catch a glimpse of something ethereal, I protect myself with only a thin layer of psychological cosmetics (*kokoro-gesō*), attempting to descend with a mind as free from worldly thoughts as possible." The cosmetics (*gesō*) are necessary, after all. When therapists try to extend beyond themselves to reach the client's mind and then return safely, they could die if they are too exposed and vulnerable. Therapists need a kind of protection.

In the *Nippon Kokugo Daijiten*[5] (2001), *kokoro-gesō*[6] is defined as, "to present oneself formally in order to make a good impression on the other. To maintain one's poise" (p. 688, our translation). In order to extend the mind further and return to the original position, one needs to become formal and poised, and to "put on" a particular feeling to a certain degree. The little prince did not have this capacity. In *The Little Prince*, the author wrote, "I even felt that nothing more fragile was to be found on this Earth" (p. 77), and "I was holding him in my arms like a child" (p. 84).

Natsuki Ikezawa says,

> To take one step further, the little prince – who came down from heaven, shared a moral message with people, was wounded in the process, and returned to heaven – is similar to Jesus Christ in terms of his behavioral patterns. If that is too strong a comparison, I would call the little prince an "angel."
>
> (p. 140, our translation)

Seen in this light, the little prince represents the bare mind itself, without awareness of being the Son of God, and before His completion as the Christ. That is also the state of just being, the intension of the *cause of existence*.

Let's take a look at *The Little Prince* in more detail.

When "I," the pilot who narrates the story, was six years old, he drew a picture of a boa constrictor swallowing and digesting an elephant; yet, adults could not understand "my masterpiece" (p. 6). They saw a hat in it. "I gave up a wonderful career as a painter." Even so,

> whenever I came across one who seemed to me at all clear-headed, I would try showing my Drawing Number One, which I have always kept by me. I wanted to find out if this was somebody with real understanding. But the answer would always be: "That is a hat." In which case I would not talk to that person about boa constrictors, or virgin forests, or stars.
>
> (p. 7)

In time, "I" became a pilot: "So I kept my own company, without anyone whom I could really talk to, until six years ago, when I made a forced landing in the Sahara desert."

The plane crashed in the Sahara desert and the repair appeared to be challenging. There was no one to offer help. There was drinking water left only for a week. It was life or death for him.

Suddenly, "I" heard a voice: "If you please – draw me a sheep!" (p. 8). It was a little boy.

"I" drew the only picture he could. The boy said, "No! no! no! I don't want an elephant inside a boa constrictor" (p. 10) – his picture was finally understood.

The picture drawn when "I" was six years of age – a boa constrictor swallowing an elephant – was a masterpiece, yet no one understood it. At the supreme life-or-death moment, a voice was heard: "If you please – draw me a sheep!" Maybe "I" was asked to draw a picture for the first time. He was asked what he really wanted for the first time. Descending to the chasm of death, "I" could finally hear that voice. And he drew what only he could draw.

You may think it is strange that a person who wanted to be a painter could only draw one picture, but it is not. There are not so many things that we want to express and can do. It may be just one thing. Didn't van Gogh want to express one thing? So did Picasso, Chagall, and Hokusai,[7] most likely.

Leiji Matsumoto,[8] a Japanese animator, always draws similar women. They are slim with big eyes, long eyelashes, and long hair. He must be able to draw other female figures with his talent, yet he continues to draw the type of female exemplified in the character of Maetel. This female figure is the one for Leiji Matsumoto. To elaborate, the Maetel-type female figure is his anima image (i.e., the feminine image within a man, or soul, in Jungian psychology). Moreover, it may be that the Japanese collective unconscious image of a woman – or more broadly speaking, the Japanese soul – is personified through this genius animator's brush. I consider this Maetel-type female image to be a continuation of Princess Kaguya,[9] who disappeared into the moon more than a thousand years ago. Sometimes an individual's expression happens to overlap with the most collective symbol. I touched upon this issue in my dissertation at the C. G. Jung Institute in Zürich, "The Disappearing Anima"; but it was rough around the edges and written over 10 years ago, so I need to refine it.

"I" drew his one image straight away at the age of six. Taking forever to complete a work, as I do, is a problem; but completing it at such a young age is also an ordeal. This is what is called the "disease of genius," and there are probably more who suffer from this disease than would be expected – hearing "that is a hat" is painful.

An image of where to go in one's life is often given in youth; it is almost like an apocalypse. Some may be able to keep it until it blooms all by itself, but in many cases, people need support to a greater or lesser extent. "I" might have become a painter if there had been someone with a little more insight, even if he or she did not guess with perfect accuracy. Unfortunately, this someone never appeared.

What is interesting here is how this misfortune allowed him to meet the little prince. *The Little Prince* could then be completed, which is now known around the world – and that is much better than his masterpiece at the age of six.

The process of a second completion after the first completion is no mean accomplishment.

Let's take a look at a Japanese movie, *A Memory* (directed by Yosihiro Nakamura, 2010), in keeping with this. The main character, Masaharu Aoyagi (played by Masato Sakai), was caught up in a national conspiracy and framed as the prime minister's assassin. He fled in desperation from such extraordinary evil. In the midst of running away, he suddenly remembered the parting words of his ex-girlfriend, Haruko Higuchi (played by Yuko Takeuchi): "I feel that we will just remain 'Good' if we continue to stay together" (our translation). In this context, "Good" refers to a stamp used in the early elementary grades. Haruko thought they could not achieve the "Excellent" stamp if they continued their relationship.

Masaharu finally got away. He even had his face surgically altered. One day, Masaharu met Haruko by chance in an elevator at the shopping mall. They both recognized each other, but no words were exchanged. Haruko had married and was with her preschool daughter and husband. After getting off the elevator, Haruko whispered to her daughter, "Stamp this onto that man's hand." What the daughter stamped onto Masaharu's hand was "Excellent."

How hard it is to go beyond "Good" to "Excellent," though. There is often a wounding that occurs along the way. In Masaharu's case, he was framed, branded a murderer, and forced to alter himself with plastic surgery. In the course of running away, however, he showed tremendous guts. As his face changed, so did his very existence. Haruko could understand the gravity of what Masaharu had accomplished in a moment's glance.

Another example is the tagline for the *Spider-Man* movie (2002): "This is my gift. It is my curse." The protagonist, Peter Parker, was bitten by a genetically engineered spider and gained special abilities (a gift). And he then had to battle against evil forces because of that ability (a curse). This tagline is actually the perfect phrase to describe the truth about the human psyche. What needs to be kept in mind, however, is that the gift and the curse[10] are inextricably linked. When these two aspects are undertaken, the "Excellent" stamp is branded, perhaps by force, upon the person. In my terminology, it is when the *disfigured hero* archetype is in a state of activation.

"I" in *The Little Prince* nearly died in the desert. A curse or wound is often required for a first completion to become a second completion. In the Introduction, this same idea was discussed in terms of "dancing with shadow" or "dancing with a wound."

I already mentioned the association of the little prince with Jesus Christ by referring to Ikezawa. In the Judeo-Christian tradition, "God saw that it was good" (Genesis 1:21, New International Version) after Creation – completion. What happened after that? Creation, which spans only a few pages at the beginning of the Bible, is followed by a long story of hardship. And then Redemption comes.

Some interpret the Creation, Fall, and Redemption as comprising one fluid narrative. If we apply this interpretation to *The Little Prince*, the protagonist's masterpiece at the age of six parallels the goodness of Creation. "I" was misunderstood for a long time, then crashed in the Sahara desert – the Fall. Finally, he could draw the second completion – the advent of a young Christ, or Redemption.

To connect this with clinical practice, some people suffer from the disease of genius (which, in fact, is quite common in childhood). No one understands them, and they reach the point of their lives being in danger. Such individuals visit a clinician, such as a psychiatrist. These clients present their suffering with all of their being. Sometimes they can explain their suffering verbally, sometimes not.

The madwoman at the shrine was one of these cases that could not be explained verbally. She was at a loss, not knowing what to say, wandering uneasily in search of the answer without knowing the question. But for just a moment, her wandering was transformed into dance. Without realizing it, she connected with her *cause of existence* and sought the answer outside of her conscious awareness. Her life would have been different if there had been more people who could have seen her movement as dance.

"I" probably couldn't explain his suffering, either. The little prince muttered what were the only appropriate words in that situation: "Draw me [a picture]" (p. 8). As soon as the little prince saw the picture, he muttered, with almost a dry tone, the correct answer that no one else had ever guessed. The picture, in which most people readily see a hat, was correctly surmised as a boa constrictor swallowing and digesting an elephant. Only a child of God can do that. A boa swallowing and digesting an elephant is what "I" had been backlogged on since the age of six. He must have been crying out with a voice no one recognized: "Please, someone, understand me."

This kind of picture determines one's entire life. An elephant is quite large. It conceals some kind of wisdom. It is slow, warm, and very strong. This good element is swallowed by a boa. The boa is about to digest this good element. A snake is often a villain in the West. When it reaches a certain size, it turns into a dragon. But in the East, a dragon is also a deity; it is therefore fearsome, but not just a villain. In the West, dragons are evil – a young man kills it and is then able to mature. A sacrifice must be made for one's individuation.[11] The boa has already surpassed the size of a snake in swallowing the elephant. The bad is swallowing and digesting the good. This is quite horrifying. It also looks like a hat. Given that a hat is worn on the head, perhaps the picture depicts what is going on in the head, i.e., a transformation of consciousness.

Whether this transformation leads to individuation or not depends on the digestive process. If the elephant's energy is strong, it could transform the boa even if the elephant is digested. In either case, swallowing and digesting something as large as an elephant is required. If this is not accomplished, "I" may have to keep living as the boa or the dragon. The picture, which no one could understand, has remained unchanged since the age of six. It stopped developing then. Digestion hasn't proceeded. Or the digestion has been feared, since nothing can be predicted once it has occurred. It may even be that "I" held the digestive process back as much as possible. This was the uneasy balance in which "I" was living. Then he finally met the little prince, who understood him. The digestive process probably started, and the boa's transformation began.

The little prince asked him to draw a sheep. This was in order to have the sheep eat baobab trees. The little prince knew that the picture "I" drew had that much power. Only someone with uniquely developed talents could breathe life into the picture. When the true genius draws, the world animates. When the true genius carves a carp, it begins to swim. This is art. The carp resides in the viewer's heart, where it moves and continues to move.

Baobab trees destroy a planet if they spread too far or grow too large. The sheep (the good) eats the baobabs (the bad); this is the opposite of the snake (the bad) eating the elephant (the good). The little prince introduces a catalyst that alters for the better the process of the boa swallowing the elephant. The little prince knew that "I" had kept that picture since the age of six. If the little prince is viewed as a young Jesus Christ, this is not surprising.

Ordinary clinicians, just like myself, cannot perform such miracles. It seems dangerous even to attempt them, but it is necessary at least to be trained not to say "hat" in the first place.

"I" did not even have the "why" question. What he had kept was the picture that no one had ever understood. This picture needed to develop for him to live this life.

The madwoman at the shrine in all likelihood – no, without doubt – also had such a picture. She could dance for just a moment with the picture. I was happy to be her audience. After 40 years, I began using the phrase, "*psycheology* that dances with madness." It seems that my picture, of the madwoman herself, had been waiting a long time to be expressed as well.

Helen Keller said,

> The task of writing an autobiography is a difficult one. When I try to classify my earliest impressions, I find that fact and fancy look alike across the years that link the past with the present. The woman paints the child's experiences in her own fantasy.
>
> (1903/2002, p. 3)

Every story may be created in the present moment.

Yet, I believe the madwoman did exist. I do not think she was just a figment of my imagination. Even if that were the case, the figment would still have its own meaning. My notion of *psycheology*, which developed from the image of "the madwoman," should not be abandoned just because it does not begin with factual accuracy. Regardless, the image of the madwoman surely exists in my mental reality. Some of you may feel that talking about mental realities simply allows writers to conjure up their own reasoning, but the most essential things exist as mental realities.

Until quite recently, the Big Bang at the beginning of the universe was estimated to have occurred about 12 billion years ago. The accepted notion today seems to be 13.7 billion years ago. The number will be corrected again. It is quite possible that an entirely different cosmology from the current one will be presented a hundred years from now. The term cosmology itself may become outdated a thousand years hence. Our consciousness desires the beginning: the Big Bang, the *Bible*, and the *Kojiki*.[12] Our unconscious seems to prepare the beginning within the range our consciousness can tolerate. If consciousness develops, a new beginning will then be prepared. The same principle applies to *psycheology*: if it advances at all, another starting point will possibly be revealed.

Though different from physical reality, mental reality must still have its own coherence, which is provided by interactions between what is conscious and what is unconscious. In the Eastern sense, it is provided by the interactions between consciousness and deep consciousness. Advanced science is no exception; it cannot get out of this interaction. Consciousness desires the beginning, and deep consciousness prepares it. The story that is created must be sufficiently coherent to be accepted. Sometimes, a genius breaks that coherence in a manner that brings consciousness a half or full step forward. This impacts the world, and human consciousness can only accept this impact within its tolerable range. If the impact is too much, it is simply passed over or ignored. In such cases, the genius' insight may lie dormant for a long time. When such an impact cannot be ignored, despite being intolerable, we experience it as madness.

The consciousness of the madwoman at the shrine was half a step out of the ordinary. Her strangeness scared and baffled people. It was not ignored. People sensed madness in it. If a viewer could step out and gain an alternate perspective, it could look completely different. I think those who lack this capacity, or do not make the effort to develop it, do not have the aptitude to be psychotherapists.

Let's continue reading *The Little Prince*. What kind of person was the little prince? The little prince's home planet was very small. "'It's a question of discipline,' the little prince informed me later on" (p. 20). "Sometimes one can safely put off what needs doing until later. But in the case of baobabs it always ends in disaster" (p. 22).

Fortunately, we live on a big planet called Earth. Earth is magnificent beyond our comprehension, and it nurtures and sustains humankind. We take Earth for granted due to its tremendous size. It is so mighty that it does not need care from us. Deforestation and global warming are debated today, but it is humanity, not Earth, that is in trouble if such conditions continue. Earth will support itself.

The little prince's planet, however, was small. It would be destroyed if not properly cared for on a daily basis. Despite living on Earth, there are many people who live on a tiny planet in terms of their mental reality. Many people with schizophrenia are like this; so was the madwoman.

It is important to continue providing tender care to the foundation every single day, as it would crack if the care were absent for even one day. It is the same with ordinary people. If care is not given every day, they do not collapse like those with schizophrenia. That is, their social adjustment does not fail entirely. If care is not given every day, however, their quality of life will deteriorate, even if they remain capable of keeping things together on the surface.

The alcoholic constellation

After the little prince left his planet, he traveled to six planets, and the seventh was Earth. There was only one man living on each of the six planets: a king on the first planet, a conceited man on the second, and a drinker on the third.

I mentioned previously that the etiological classification in psychiatry involves the psychogenic cause, the endogenous cause, and the exogenous cause. And to add to it, I discussed the necessity of the *cause of existence.* The case of the fiancée's death, provided by Hayao Kawai, corresponds to the psychogenic cause, and the madwoman at the shrine corresponds to the endogenous cause.

Now that the drinker has come up, I will discuss alcoholism as an example of the exogenous cause. We must know that dependence, not just alcoholism, is an important phenomenon when considering existence and madness.

The drinker had been drinking.

> "'I'm drinking," said the drinker, with a mournful air.
> "Why are you drinking?" asked the little prince.
> "To forget," replied the drinker.
> "To forget what?" inquired the little prince, who was already starting to feel sorry for him.
> "To forget that I'm ashamed," confessed the drinker, hanging his head.
> "Ashamed of what?" persisted the little prince, who wanted to help him.
> "Ashamed of drinking!" concluded the drinker, retreating into permanent silence.
>
> (p. 42)

Those who are becoming, or have already become, alcoholics must continue abstinence as a daily activity and "care." Failing in this care, their daily living becomes horribly rough. More likely, it will not be long before their very lives are in danger.

Alcohol dependence is one of the most dreadful diseases in the mental health field. Such people only live to be about 50 years old, and the process of dying is truly miserable. Abandoned by family and having lost their jobs, they nevertheless continue drinking, which brings on the physical wreckage. Finally, death arrives as if it were an extended suicide.

The dialogue between the drinker and the little prince shows the primary pathology of alcohol dependence quite well. The drinker drinks to forget and shuts himself up, so that his own space becomes smaller and smaller. Over time, the alcoholic's sense of self screams as if squished and squeezed, and then dies off. A truly horrifying disease.

It would appear that one of the devil's projects is to deprive people's souls. "The Bottle Imp" by Robert Louis Stevenson, the famed author of *Treasure Island* and "The Strange Case of Dr. Jekyll and Mr. Hyde," is a powerful short story on this theme. At the end, an alcoholic man appears whose decline is chilling and disturbing.

Keawe is a sailor. He encounters a magic bottle, which makes any dream come true. A very ugly imp lives inside the bottle and grants anything the current owner wants. As the owner of the bottle explains:

> There is one thing the imp cannot do – he cannot prolong life; and, it would not be fair to conceal from you, there is a drawback to the bottle; for if a man die before he sells it, he must burn in hell forever. . . . but it cannot be sold at all, unless at a loss. If you sell it for as much as you paid for it, back it comes to you again like a homing pigeon.
>
> (1891/2013, pp. 334–335)

Keawe buys the bottle, and as the story progresses, his wife ends up buying it for three centimes. It is difficult to sell the bottle for two centimes. The subsequent owner has to buy it for a centime, sell it to another, and then . . . However, a drinker buys the bottle from Keawe's wife so that he can drink. The man says that it will be a good bottle to take to hell, such that he would not sell it for a centime. The story ends with him walking away with the bottle.

The drinker knew his soul would be sent to hell, so he bought the bottle to at least continue drinking in this world. "I reckon I'm going anyway," he says (p. 358). Dependence is that horrendous. This is just a story, but it portrays accurately how someone who is substance-dependent will knowingly go even to the gates of hell.

Generally, it is difficult for the alcohol-dependent person to cut down, so quitting alcohol is the only way to treat the condition. In the traditional Japanese arts, there are a few works that depict alcohol dependence. There is *Shibahama* in *Rakugo*, and *Shibahama-no-Kawazaifu* in *Kabuki*.[13] The scenarios presented are almost identical: a fish merchant (the alcoholic) quits drinking and recovers with the support of his wife. But the conclusions are different. In *Rakugo*, his wife rewards the man, saying, "You have been working very hard without any alcohol for three years. Please have a glass"

(Iijima, 1998, p. 87, our translation) – but he rejects it. In *Kabuki*, however, the man accepts the offer. From the mental health perspective, the *Rakugo* version is correct. If these individuals can quit drinking for three years, there is a high chance they will be able to continue their abstinence for the rest of their lives. However, even if they are abstinent for three years, just a sip will gradually lead the person to consume more and more, and they will return to the old pattern. If those who have been successfully abstinent emulate the fish merchant's attitude after watching the *Kabuki* version, the outcome will be tragic. I realize it is a big favor to ask, but as a huge fan of *Kabuki*, I would like people involved with the form to consider a creative alternative to this ending.

Being able to enjoy only an appropriate amount of alcohol is difficult for people of a certain constitution (whose foundation is very similar to someone with a biological vulnerability towards personhood disorder; they share the pathology of pursuing godhood unconsciously, as mentioned previously). People with a physiological disposition develop a tendency to go too far, e.g., drinking before work. Their body becomes weaker and weaker, they become violent, and they are often hospitalized. In mental health, alcohol (the exogenous cause) is first considered as the primary cause (of the dependency). Next, the relationship clients have to alcohol, the circumstances surrounding them, and the like are taken into consideration. An attempt is made to discover the solution by analyzing the situation that drove them to dependence. Clinicians try to grasp what is happening to such clients in a holistic context, including the clients themselves, their families, and their work environments. Clinicians attempt to locate such clients as the star around which alcohol dependence has constellated.

Yet, these clients cannot escape the question, "Why? Why me and not others?" Those who are consumed by this question will drink themselves to death.

In such a situation, an attitude of looking at the *cause of existence* can be useful. That is, psychotherapists try to find a constellation that also includes the "why" questions. When therapists express curiosity about why something has come to pass (which is often overlooked), a glimmer may appear. If they stay attuned to the glimmer, it first appears like a fog and then gradually takes shape. If it continues developing, therapists sometimes catch a momentary but clear glimpse of the constellation hidden in the depths. Sometimes it is beautiful, sometimes not. Beauty and ugliness are simply mirror images of each other. There is an extraordinary coexistence of the divine and the demonic in such a deep constellation, which includes the "why" questions. While such coexistence turns into a front-and-back-relationship (Jekyll and Hyde) in the West, it is a harmonious combination in the East, especially in Japan.

When the constellation begins to dance in the depths, sometimes it looks very beautiful, and sometimes very ugly. Yet, it is somehow breathtaking when taken altogether. Such beauty can be hard to understand, so here are some examples.

One is from a Japanese *manga* and another is from a Japanese TV drama.

The first example is *Star of the Giants*,[14] a Japanese *manga* written by Ikki Kajiwara and illustrated by Noboru Kawasaki (*Shōnen Weekly Magazine*, 1966–1971). When Hyūma was little, Ittetsu got drunk, and in a fit of anger, hit Hyūma and flipped a table. What Ittetsu did to Hyūma was terrible. Now, however, Ittetsu is a radiant part of the constellation surrounding him, both for Hyūma and the readers.

This harmonious dance can also be seen as a different constellation if viewed from another perspective. If Ittetsu is seen as the primary star, he tossed the table with every fiber of his being. It was ugly, but he was dancing with all the determination and hope that he could muster in that extreme moment. Hyūma, who sensed his father's heart; Hyūma's sister, Akiko; and Ittetsu's now-deceased wife all came to accept his behaviors as part of the development of Ittetsu's dance. In a case such as the drinker in "The Bottle Imp," who bought the bottle for two centimes, it is impossible to sense his constellation with any depth. This is because no pain, effort, or conflict is experienced. Conflict and anguish are the keys to the constellation, the dance, and the *cause of existence*.

The second example is *The Queen's Classroom*[15] (2005–2006, Nippon Television), a Japanese TV drama written by Kazuhiko Yukawa. The protagonist, Maya Akutsu (starring Yuuki Amami), was an unremarkable elementary school[16] teacher who was kind to her students. She was falsely accused of abusing a student, and quit her job. She got married, lost her son in an accident, and divorced. She intended to commit suicide, but in learning that a former student had attempted suicide, decided to return to teaching instead. At the second elementary school, she was attacked by a student with a box cutter and nearly died from a stab to the chest. In the course of these events, she had become the true Maya Akutsu. Despite the students at her third school considering her a devil, she became a teacher who guided and developed her students, no matter what the cost. She challenged them to wake up to the realities facing them, even at the risk of being seen as cruel and sent to the re-education center for teachers a second time.

Maya was already connected to her *cause of existence*. She recognized the cause of her existence. She lived with it. She lived the cruelest yet most fulfilling life through her *cause of existence*. This drama is masterful in depicting the transition from "White Maya" to "Gray Maya" to "Black Maya."[17]

Myōe, a Buddhist saint from the Kamakura Period,[18] cut off his own ear in order to gain the true religious spirit. It is often necessary to become wounded in order to place oneself in the constellation that includes the *cause of existence*. It is as though the wound's existence opens up that of the individual.

Notes

1 Translators' note: In the original Japanese, the words used to describe the individuals are gender-neutral, such that the quote could be referring to either a man or a woman losing a partner in either a heterosexual or homosexual relationship.
2 Translators' note: Intension is a term used in logic and signifies "the internal quantity or content of a notion or concept, the sum of the attributes contained in it; the number of qualities connoted by a term" ("Intension," 2016).
3 Translators' note: The passage is suggesting that what was initially a distracted glance towards the mountains ended up providing Guggenbühl-Craig with a flash of insight regarding his "why" questions.
4 Translators' note: The notion of requiring some level of presentation and/or protection to avoid excessive vulnerability is a common one in depth psychology. One example would be Jung's concept of "persona," which itself derives from the ancient Greeks' use of masks in the theater.
5 Translators' note: A Japanese-language dictionary.
6 Translators' note: *Kokoro*: mind; *gesō*: cosmetics.
7 Translators' note: Katsushika Hokusai (1760–1849) was a Japanese artist, *ukiyo-e* (woodblock) painter and printmaker of the Edo period (1603–1868). He is best known for the woodblock print series, *Thirty-six Views of Mount Fuji* (c. 1831), which includes the famous "Great Wave off Kanagawa."
8 Translators' note: 1938–
9 Translators' note: From *The Tale of the Bamboo-Cutter*, the oldest Japanese narrative.
10 Translators' note: While a gift (god) is generally followed by a curse (devil) in the West, the order is often reversed in Japan. For instance, a Japanese monster appears first, and Ultraman (a heroic character in a Japanese television series) appears next to combat the monster.
11 Translators' note: The element sacrificed may be either bad, like the snake/dragon; or good, as with the elephant.
12 Translators' note: *The Record of Ancient Matters*, written in 714, known as the oldest Japanese record of history and mythology.
13 Translators' note: See endnote in Preface [English Edition] for descriptions of *Rakugo* and *Kabuki*.
14 Translators' note: *Star of the Giants* is a Japanese *manga* about a son (Hyūma Hoshi) who receives grueling baseball training from his father (Ittetsu), and goes on to play for the Yomiuri Giants (professional baseball) team. In his day, Ittetsu was himself a legendary third baseman for the Yomiuri Giants. After retiring from the league, Ittetsu struggled to move on with his life, working as a laborer to support his family by day, and drinking heavily by night. When Ittetsu's wife passed away, however, he dedicated himself to training his son, Hyūma, to be a great baseball player like himself. Hyūma initially hated his father and the grueling training, but awakened to the joy of playing baseball as he grew older. Eventually, Hyūma told his father that he was determined to play for the Yomiuri Giants. Ittetsu pointed to the evening star, Hesperus, and likened it to the "Star of the Giants." He encouraged Hyūma to become the star of the Yomiuri Giants, and resolved not to drink again until that day came.

In Japanese, the word *hoshi* – Ittetsu and Hyūma's surname – signifies a star in the sky.
15 Translators' note: *The Queen's Classroom* is a classroom drama depicting a hard-edged teacher and her students.
16 Translators' note: In Japan, elementary school runs through the equivalent of sixth grade in the American system, or ages 11–12.

17 Translators' note: At her first school, Maya was a sweet, angelic teacher who always put a smile on her face. She tried to be a good teacher, engaging with her students like a friend. This approach worked against her, however, generating a sense of opposition in her students. Back then, she was dressed in white and her hair waved freely (White Maya).

At the next school, Maya was tougher on her students, but was still in a process of transition. Her outfits consisted primarily of gray suits, with her hair in a ponytail, as if to symbolize her transition (Gray Maya).

In her third classroom – the one depicted in the TV show – Maya presents her students with a challenging wall to scale, endeavoring to awaken them to the reality of needing to make every effort to overcome the real-world challenges in their lives. Maya always wears a black turtleneck, probably an attempt to cover the big scar on her chest (from the knife attack at the second school), and pulls her hair back in a bun (Black Maya).

18 Translators' note: 1185–1333.

References

Akita, I. (2000). Henro-to-sonzai-in [Pilgrimage and the *cause of existence*]. *Psyche, 19*, 120–127.

Christie, A. (1944). *Towards zero*. London, England: Harper Collins Publishers.

Descartes, R. (1952). Discourse on the method of rightly conducting the reason and seeking for truth in the sciences. In R. M. Hutchins (Series Ed.), *Great books of the western world* (Vol. 31, E. S. Haldane & G. R. T. Ross, Trans, pp. 41–67). Chicago, IL: Encyclopædia Britannica. (Original work published 1637)

Iijima, T. (Ed.) (1998). Shibahama (performed by M. Katsura). In M. Anno, T. Mori, H. Inoue, & O. Ikeuchi (Eds.), *Chikuma bungaku-no-mori: Kokoro-arawareru-hanashi* [Chikuma Press literature collection: Stories to freshen the heart] (Vol. 2, pp. 59–88). Tokyo, Japan: Chikuma Shobo.

Intension. (2016). *In Oxford English dictionary*. Retrieved from http://www.oed.com

Kawai, H. (1967). *Jung shinrigaku nyūmon* [Introduction to Jungian psychology]. Tokyo, Japan: Baifukan.

Keller, H. (2002). *The story of my life*. New York, NY: New American Library. (Original work published 1903)

Kokoro-gesō. (2001). In Shogakukan Kokugo Jiten Henshubu (Ed.), *Nihon kokugo daijiten* [Japanese dictionary] (2nd ed., Vol. 5). Tokyo, Japan: Shogakukan.

Saint-Exupéry, A. de (2000). *The little prince and letter to a hostage* (T. V. F. Cuffe, Trans.). London, England: Penguin Books. (Original work published 1943)

Stevenson, R. L. (2013). The bottle imp. In D. Sander & J. Weisman (Eds.), *The treasury of the fantastic* (pp. 332–358). San Francisco, CA: Tachyon. (Original work published 1891)

Chapter 2

What is madness?

Mental disorders and madness

Several presumably alcohol-dependent characters appeared in Chapter 1: the man near my childhood home; the drinker in *The Little Prince*; the last person to purchase the bottle in "The Bottle Imp"; and the fisherman husband who featured in both the *Rakugo* story, *Shibahama,* and the *Kabuki* play, *Shibahama-no-Kawazaifu*.

The clinical conditions that practitioners observe in alcohol dependence and personhood disorders closely resemble each other in their essences. The inability to stop drinking heavily in alcohol-dependent individuals leads to damage of body, mind, even soul – and eventually leads to their deaths. While the process of damaging themselves cannot be described as simply for those with borderline personality disorder, for example, they tend to panic in response to trivial affairs, often leading to repeated wrist-cutting or overdoses. I will discuss this issue later, but the common factor in these two clinical conditions is that the individuals in question get out of order in "personhood" (*jin-kaku*)[1] due to a pursuit of "godhood" (*shin-kaku*),[2] whether consciously or unconsciously. Once alcohol-dependent people become drunk, they speak and act like God or the devil. When sober, they are ordinary, calm, kind-hearted citizens; yet the dynamic at the depth of their psyches is presumably a conflict over godhood and personhood.

The drinker in *The Little Prince* was ashamed of drinking. As he could not stop drinking, he was even more ashamed of himself. He kept drinking to forget his shame, and ended up "retreating into permanent silence" (1943/2000, p. 42). The drinker in "The Bottle Imp" did not experience any conflict, as he was not bothered about whether he would be sent to hell. He was content so long as he could drink in the moment. When an attitude is so thoroughly held, it may give a helping hand to others. The drinker helped Keawe and his wife, who were desperate. The fisherman in *Shibahama* and *Shibahama-no-Kawazaifu* could recover himself with the support of his wife's wits and devotion, though the endings were different.

There is, however, a short story that depicts a dreadful situation: "The Black Cat," written by Edgar Allan Poe.

> From my infancy I was noted for the docility and humanity of my disposition. My tenderness of heart was even so conspicuous as to make me the jest of my companions. I was especially fond of animals . . . We had birds, goldfish, a fine dog, rabbits, a small monkey, and *a cat.*
>
> This latter was a remarkably large and beautiful animal, entirely black, and sagacious to an astonishing degree . . .
>
> Pluto – this was the cat's name . . .
>
> Our friendship lasted, in this manner, for several years, during which my general temperament and character – through the instrumentality of the Fiend Intemperance – had (I blush to confess it) experienced a radical alteration for the worse. I grew, day by day, more moody, more irritable, more regardless of the feelings of others. I suffered myself to use intemperate language to my wife. At length, I even offered her personal violence . . . But my disease grew upon me – for what disease like Alcohol! – and at length even Pluto, who was now becoming old, and consequently somewhat peevish – even Pluto began to experience the effects of my ill temper.
>
> One night, returning home, much intoxicated, from one of my haunts about town . . . [Pluto] inflicted a slight wound upon my hand with his teeth . . . A more than fiendish malevolence, gin-nurtured, thrilled every fiber of my frame. I took from my waistcoat-pocket a penknife, opened it, grasped the poor beast by the throat, and deliberately cut one of its eyes from the socket!
>
> . . . I experienced a sentiment half of horror, half of remorse, for the crime of which I had been guilty; but it was, at best, a feeble and equivocal feeling, and the soul remained untouched.
>
> . . . And then came, as if to my final and irrevocable overthrow, the spirit of PERVERSENESS. Of this spirit philosophy takes no account. Yet I am not more sure that my soul lives, than I am that perverseness is one of the primitive impulses of the human heart – one of the indivisible primary faculties, or sentiments, which give direction to the character of Man. Who has not, a hundred times, found himself committing a vile or a stupid action, for no other reason than because he knows he should *not*? . . . It was this unfathomable longing of the soul *to vex itself* – to offer violence to its own nature – to do wrong for the wrong's sake only – that urged me to continue and finally to consummate the injury I had inflicted upon the unoffending brute. One morning, in cold blood, I slipped a noose about its neck and hung it to the limb of a tree; – hung it with the tears streaming from my eyes, and with the bitterest remorse at my heart; – hung it *because* I knew that it had loved me, and *because* I felt it had given me no reason of offense; – hung it *because* I knew that in so doing I was committing a sin.
>
> (1843/2002, pp. 203–205)

Subsequently, he split his wife's head with an ax, and his murder was eventually exposed.

It really is a story full of horror, which is unmerciful in describing the terrors of alcohol dependency, personhood disorders, and psychopathy. As alcohol dependence proceeds, an individual's personhood becomes disordered little by little, and the state of personhood disorder follows. Beyond this, a person will enter the state of psychopathy, as if his or her human mind had been totally lost. What could be more frightening than this disease?

There are various stages leading towards alcohol dependency, though each case is ultimately unique to the individual. Some, for instance, show atypical drunkenness suddenly. While the stages are not always accurate, then, most often they take the following course: a condition in which the individuals enjoy drinking a moderate amount of alcohol; a stage where no particular problem appears, though the amount of alcohol consumption is rather too much; and a stage in which their social adjustment remains while some problems occur. If they step over this final line, they will become alcohol-dependent. The definition of alcohol dependency varies, but to put it simply, it is a condition in which people cannot stop themselves despite reaching a point where they must.

In "The Black Cat," this line was crossed. It is full of language about evil; the main character, for example, was cruel enough to be described as fiendish. The man had been "noted for the docility and humanity of [his] disposition" (p. 203), but alcohol gradually led to this change in his personality (Figure 2.1).

While human nature is generally recognized to be fairly stable, it can flip over in a situation like this.

When excessive kindness is expressed externally, the cruelty of which all humans are capable sinks down into the internal world. Cruelty eventually develops beyond the control of the ego and gains autonomy. In ordinary circumstances, the ego maintains a balance between kindness and cruelty: kindness – ego – cruelty. But superhuman kindness, like an angel, cannot be controlled by the ego. Some cue gets triggered, and it flips over. In the case of "The Black Cat," the trigger was alcohol.

On the other hand, some cases do not flip over. This happens when there is a modest spirit of self-sacrifice. Modest kindness – which is not "so conspicuous as to make [one] the jest of [one's] companions" – and a spirit of self-sacrifice can serve as a "protective suit" or "psychological cosmetics" (*kokoro-gesō*). Evil cannot act autonomously in the face of this spirit of self-sacrifice, though it tries. It is the same composition of powerlessness the devil faces with Jesus Christ.

If a flesh-and-blood human attempts to be overly self-sacrificing, the risk for the kinds of events depicted in "The Black Cat" increases. The protagonist

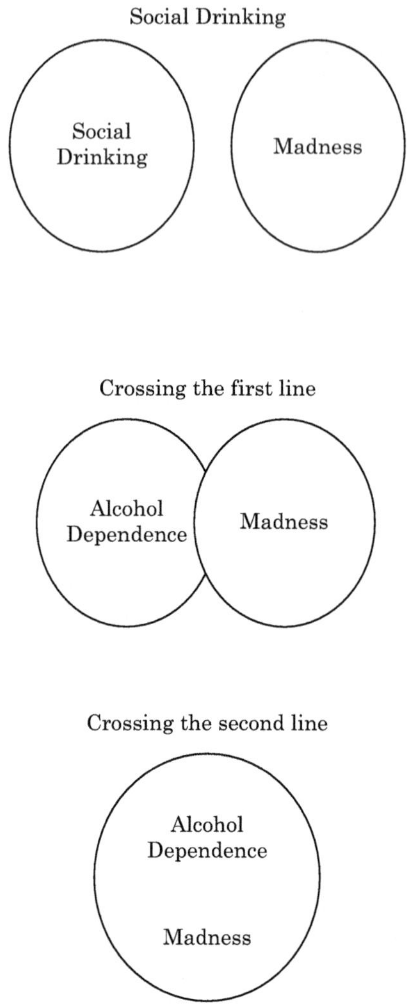

Figure 2.1

of "The Black Cat" probably had a Christ-like quality. While Jesus Christ blossomed through asceticism and abstinence, however, the man in "The Black Cat" wilted under the influence of the devil and drinking. It is better for normal people to stick with a modest spirit of self-sacrifice.

Meeting the black cat was fine. It was not a big deal whether it was white or black. However, the protagonist named the black cat Pluto, King of the Underworld. Spooky images of witches, which often feature black cats, also come to mind. He invited Pluto into his world. Everything has hidden potential. The mission of the black cat was oriented by its name, which is to say that the black cat's mission was determined when the name was given.

The word *meishin* ("superstition")[3] is recognized as fallacy nowadays, as science has progressed remarkably in this modern age (ours is nevertheless an archaic age if we imagine what will be a thousand years hence). *Meishin* is being abandoned by today's collective consciousness, but it still lives deep in the human psyche. It can be defined as believing in heaven or the afterworld, or as a belief that is false and irrational. *Meishin* is also a path to something unworldly. It is something faintly anticipated and intuited, although not understandable or explainable in conscious, verbal terms. It nevertheless contains something valuable that should not be abandoned just because it is unexplainable with our present understanding. What begins with only faint anticipation and intuition often yields to conscious, verbal articulation in time.

I mentioned that one becomes alcohol-dependent if a certain line is crossed, and the condition that arises in crossing the second line is described in "The Black Cat." When this Pluto, King of the Underworld, is invited in, one begins to engage in superhuman devilry; this state is described as "psychopathy" in mental health. In "The Black Cat," Poe's mind extended beyond alcoholism (which affects the body and mind) to psychopathy (which affects the soul). At the level of psychopathy, one becomes more sensitized to faint anticipations and intuitions, while abandoning them at the same time.

Mental disorders are not equal to madness. When this second line is crossed, however, mental disorders (in this case, alcohol dependency) overlap with madness. The man in "The Black Cat" gouged Pluto's eye out with a knife, killed it by hanging, and murdered his wife by splitting her head with an axe. Heavy drinking caused him to cross the first line and he became alcohol-dependent. He subsequently crossed the second line and became psychopathic – that is madness.

In Poe's language, it is "the spirit of perverseness" that triggers one to cross the second line. It is a "primitive impulse" and the "unfathomable longing of the soul *to vex itself* – to offer violence to its own nature – to do wrong for the wrong's sake only" (p. 204). People with this attribute are called devils. The word "perverse" is derived from the Latin *pervertus* ("flipped over"), meaning that one wanders[4] from the right path.

The "right path" is the path shown by God. People who are considered to have wandered from that path are deemed perverse and degenerate. This is extremely important in thinking about the nature of Western mental health. B. A. Morel's degeneration theory swept Europe around the late 19th century, mainly in the 1880s; but in my estimation, it remains the central tenant supporting contemporary mental health.

When the second line is crossed, the power "to offer violence to [one's] own nature" (p. 204) and for the mind "to do wrong for the wrong's sake only" become activated. A change in the soul's quality takes place, so to speak – a condition well depicted in "The Black Cat."

Psychopathy

"Psychopathy" originated as a psychiatric term. It is also used in daily life to describe brutal criminals, though this usage is not as common in Japan. Hannibal Lecter in *The Silence of the Lambs*, an American movie released in 1991, provides a representative image of psychopathy. He was so bloodthirsty that I even hesitate to depict him here. As an alternative, I would like to introduce a case by Carl Gustav Jung (1875–1961), the founder of analytical psychology.

> A young woman had been admitted to the hospital, suffering from "melancholia." . . . The diagnosis was schizophrenia, or "dementia praecox," in the phrase of those days. The prognosis: poor.
>
> This woman happened to be in my section. At first I did not dare to question the diagnosis . . . And yet the case struck me as strange. I had the feeling that it was not a matter of schizophrenia but of ordinary depression, and resolved to apply my own method. At the time I was much occupied with diagnostic association studies, and so I undertook an association experiment with the patient. In addition, I discussed her dreams with her. In this way I succeeded in uncovering her past, which the anamnesis had not clarified. I obtained information directly from the unconscious, and this information revealed a dark and tragic story.
>
> Before the woman married she had known a man, the son of a wealthy industrialist, in whom all the girls of the neighborhood were interested. Since she was very pretty, she thought her chances of catching him were fairly good. But apparently he did not care for her, and so she married another man.
>
> Five years later an old friend visited her. They were talking over old times, and he said to her, "When you got married it was quite a shock to someone – your Mr. X" (the wealthy industrialist's son) . . . Her depression dated from this period, and several weeks later led to a catastrophe. She was bathing her children, first her four-year-old daughter and then her two-year-old son. She lived in a country where the water supply was not perfectly hygienic; there was pure spring water for drinking and tainted water from the river for bathing and washing. While she was bathing the little girl, she saw the child sucking at the sponge, but did not stop her. She even gave her little son a glass

> of the impure water to drink. Naturally, she did this unconsciously, or only half-consciously, for her mind was already under the shadow of the incipient depression.
>
> A short time later, after the incubation period had passed, the girl came down with typhoid fever and died. The girl had been her favorite. The boy was not infected. At that moment the depression reached its acute stage, and the woman was sent to the institution.
>
> From the association test I had seen that she was a murderess, and I had learned many of the details of her secret. It was at once apparent that this was a sufficient reason for her depression. Essentially, it was a psychogenic disturbance and not a case of schizophrenia.
>
> (1962/1989, pp. 115–117)

This woman, diagnosed with schizophrenia (which was *dementia praecox* back then), became a client of Jung's towards the beginning of his career. Jung assessed her as having psychogenic depression and discovered her past through an association experiment and dream analysis. He "obtained information directly from the unconscious," which "revealed a dark and tragic story" (p. 115). After some indecision, he shared the facts with her. "And it was tragic for the patient to have to listen to it and accept it. But the result was that in two weeks it proved possible to discharge her, and she was never again institutionalized" (p. 116).

Jung thought he grasped the essence of this case by knowing the dark and tragic story. And he thought that she was cured because she accepted it (or brought it up into consciousness). I don't think Jung's understanding was wrong, but another perspective might be possible if we place the emphasis on a different aspect.

This client killed her daughter, though she did so unconsciously. She crossed the second line at that time. This was the appearance of psychopathy, at which point madness descended upon her. Jung discovered her path to murder and weighed it heavily in his mind. He might have felt satisfied because he unraveled the case, which no one had been able to understand, using his own method of word association in conjunction with dream analysis. Jung understood the case, the client accepted the fact, her depression disappeared, and she was never institutionalized again – it was truly something to celebrate. But how should we understand the true, albeit temporary, madness that had descended upon her? That is the most difficult question this case poses to me, and indeed, to all humankind.

> When she was discharged, she departed bearing her heavy burden. She *had* to bear this burden. The loss of the child had been frightful for her, and her expiation had already begun with the depression and her confinement to the institution.
>
> (p. 117)

I totally agree with Jung's philosophy of treatment: "bearing one's cross." Doing so offers the power to transform oneself, and the *disfigured hero* is an extension that builds upon this foundation (Akita, 2001).

Although what Jung described here was truly respectful, he did not mention the fact or discuss the meaning of psychopathy having dominated the client's body and mind, albeit briefly. She killed her own daughter. At that moment, she was mad. This is madness. It is this point that should be raised first in this case.

Schizophrenia and depression are terms in mental health, not in madness. When the client killed her daughter, she might not have been mentally disordered, but she was mad. By the time she was institutionalized, she had definitely reached the state of mental disorder, but it was not quite clear whether she remained in a state of madness. She was no longer mentally disordered when the treatment ended, but it is unclear with the madness.

In this case, Jung saw her sin as the main problem, and imposed upon the client to bear her burden. Did she bear the burden, then? I cannot compare to Jung, but in my clinical experience, when an overly heavy burden is borne, a person has difficulty moving forward. At the same time, moving forward is the only "treatment." If she began to move forward in only two weeks, however, a big problem remains. It is possible that the psychopathy continued to dominate her, despite a lack of telltale incidents or symptoms on the surface. In other words, it remains a mystery whether she achieved individuation in the depths of her soul.

This client could not achieve the love she originally wanted. She was destined to marry another man and have two children. After five years of marriage, when the conversation with her old friend brought her the feeling that she might have been able to achieve her original love, the "devil" showed up – psychopathy appeared. This was the essence of her pathology. Who would ever think that her friend's conversation would be the whispering of the devil? You can decide for yourself whether to see the friend's conversation as the devil's whispers or not. While holding that feeling of regret within herself, she could have enriched the memory of her younger days more colorfully, and expressed it all in her attractive smile.

But she did not have enough resolve to resist the whispering. No matter how strong the conflict that comes up, one normally will not do such a thing, even unconsciously. The "unfathomable longing of the soul *to vex itself* – to offer violence to its own nature – to do wrong for the wrong's sake only" (Poe, 1843/2002, p. 204) appeared in this woman.

What was essential in this case was not just to assess her as having psychogenic depression. It was not just to find out the untold story behind it, either. The devil would surely whisper to her again. The question would be how her heart would react to it then – that should be the essence of this case. It is possible that Jung's treatment might have touched upon this essence, and he just did not depict it. Even so, I still wanted him to mention it, considering that the appearance of psychopathy is the very target at which Western mental health takes heavy aim.

The devil is undoubtedly projected onto the terms "degeneration" and "psychopathy." These two ideas were hotly debated at the dawn of psychiatric medicine. It is quite rare for them to be discussed in psychiatric symptomatology today, however, perhaps in an attempt to expunge explicit religious tones. To me, the ultimate mission of Western mental health is to contain the devil. While its manifestation is very different, I perceive the same grounding in Christianity.[5] In my mind, the clinician's initial role might have been to exorcise the devil. At some point, a more suitable exorcist must have been demanded, giving rise to a new era.

To return to Jung's case, the client unconsciously committed a crime that could be deemed murder. The bearing of responsibility is the most important issue. This relates to the question of whether to find her not guilty or to reduce her penalty for a crime that occurred unconsciously, i.e., outside her ego's control, at the mercy of the secret of which even she was not conscious. In other words, was she insane or diminished in capacity?

It is also a matter of where to position the subject that causes sin: the ego or one's whole existence. If the ego is considered to be central, it is no wonder that a misdoing would not be blamed if it happened when the ego was out of control.

This attitude may be suitable for the Western psyche, which demands a strong ego as a sign of maturity. The Western ego is really strong, though strong in the Western sense. In Europe, though there are wide differences between countries, a baby is generally considered to be an individual who has a unique personality from birth. In providing a separate room for the baby, the mother demands and expects that the baby cry to let the mother know when it is hungry. Raised in such a manner from birth, by the age of five or six, Western kids are quite different from Japanese kids of the same age. They sometimes make facial expressions that are almost identical to those of adults. Of course, they don't have the abilities of an adult; but their eyes are claiming that they are individuals with unique personalities, and not such beings as would readily allow interference from others. To me as a Japanese person, such eyes are far from likable, yet they insist on who they are to the fullest extent. They are like lion cubs threatening other animals with all their might. Given that they will grow up to be regal adult lions, the mightiness of their egos is not comparable to that of the Japanese.

I wrote "when the ego [is] out of control," but how the ego comes to be out of control varies. There is no end of examples, from the rage in response to the sudden breakup with a loved one, to the betrayal of your best friend, to being deceived. Suffering from mental disorders is also an example. There can be a state in which one loses the ego's control, even though no psychotic symptoms are apparent, whether due to heartbreak, betrayal, or deception. Yet in criminal cases such as murder, only a mental health evaluation is given – only mental "diseases" are assessed. When a paranoid hallucination is due to schizophrenia and the ego is out of control, the crime is typically not charged based on a lack of mental capacity.

As mentioned before, however, a state of mental disorder is not the only thing that can happen when the ego's control is lost. A murderer experiences madness at the moment of the crime (though I have never actually witnessed a murder scene). Madness can be momentary or chronic. In any case, only considering someone to be lacking in mental capacity if his or her madness is manifested in a psychotic manner is totally defective. If a murderer says, "I killed the person because I was in a rage," and he was not at the level of a psychotic state, he would not have a chance to be exculpated. But he was outside the ego's control when he was in a rage. There are times when the degree of lost control is about the same as that in a psychotic state. Who can say that the momentary madness of a rage is less mad than a paranoid hallucination caused by a psychotic state? You can see how narrow and shallow our perception of madness is.

It is very hard to grasp the essence of madness. Nevertheless, we must have some countermeasures against it. Psychiatric medicine is supposed to be our primary one, but psychiatrists' specialty is to help people who are unable to adapt to society or people who are distressed. Anything beyond these is outside their expertise, at the least. Psychiatric medicine is firmly medicine, and is not *psycheology* (Akita, 2002, p. 26).

There is no other field besides psychiatric medicine that we can rely upon at present, but the judicial system's overdependence on it these days is still intolerable. This overdependence is one of our modern diseases.

To avoid misunderstanding, let me recapitulate briefly here. Regarding mental capacity, cultural differences must be considered when questioning where to position the subject who causes sin: the ego or one's whole existence. On the other hand, the issue of losing one's ego control, which is not limited to the psychotic state, is so universal that it transcends cultural differences.

The beauty of Snow-white and the Queen

As "The Black Cat" was a short story written by an individual, I would now like to pick up a story from folklore to continue the discussion.

The first edition of *Grimm's Fairy Tales* was published in 1812, and went through several editions, up to the seventh – the classical edition – which was published in 1857. If we include the Ölenberg manuscript, which was written before the initial print, there are eight editions. In Japan, it is truly fortunate that the Ölenberg manuscript, the first edition, the second edition, and the seventh edition have all been translated.

What I would like to cover here is "Little Snow-White," which is one of the most famous fairy tales in *Grimm's Fairy Tales*. It will allow us to see how psychopathy is depicted in a fairy tale. To describe psychopathy in a phrase, it is a state in which one totally lacks a human heart. The psychopath commits an atrocity as if nothing were wrong. The main character in "The Black Cat" reached this state of psychopathy, which is one form of madness, by crossing the first line and then the second line; and in Jung's case, too, it can be said that psychopathy must have appeared instantaneously.

As I imagine few are unfamiliar with the story of "Little Snow-White," I will skip a description of the story, but it is important to note that there was no stepmother depicted in the Ölenberg manuscript and initial print versions of the story. The one who tried to kill Snow-white was her biological mother. After the second edition, however, the story changed to one in which the biological mother died right after giving birth to Snow-white, and the stepmother, who was the second wife, tried to kill Snow-white (Grimm & Grimm, 1812/2014, 1857/1983). The biological mother trying to kill her own daughter is too cruel. However, it becomes easier for readers, especially children, to accept this cruelty if it is a stepmother. That was the reason for the change, which is the same reason why there are many stories in which a stepmother bullies or kills a child in folktales. So the image of the stepmother as a bad mother has been fixed. In reality, it is a pity for stepmothers; this is one of the sins brought on by folktales.

Folktales depict what is happening in the depths of the human psyche; you should not directly apply it to reality as it is written. Rather, it is better used as a means of knowing what is going on in our psyches.

No significant change was found between editions of "Little Snow-White" beyond that of the birth mother changing to the stepmother. This stepmother was believed to be stunningly beautiful, so whenever the magic looking-glass was asked who was the fairest of them all, it would answer, "Thou, O Queen, art the fairest of all!" (1857/1983, p. 250) When Snow-white turned seven years old, however, she became far fairer than her stepmother.

> And once when the Queen asked her looking-glass:
>
> "Looking-glass, Looking-glass, on the wall,
> Who in this land is the fairest of all?"
>
> it answered:
>
> "Thou art fairer than all who are here, Lady Queen,
> But more beautiful still is Snow-white, as I ween."
>
> (p. 250)

Everyone knows this scene; it may be the most famous scene in human history. In the Bible, there are many famous scenes, such as Eve eating an apple when tempted by the Serpent, Noah's ark, the crucifixion of Christ, and so forth. Greek mythology also has numerous famous scenes, although they do not evoke instantaneous images to the same degree. There are many famous scenes other than myths, like Don Quixote diving into windmills, Raskolnikov killing the old lady with an ax, and so on.

There are also many famous scenes in "Little Snow-White" besides the scene of the magic looking-glass: Snow-white and the seven dwarfs living happily together, Snow-white choked on an apple and struck down, and Snow-white awakening with the Prince's kiss (this scene was added in the later revisions, and was not written in the original version of *Grimm's Fairy Tales*). I would say that "Little Snow-White" is the masterpiece of the narrative category in terms of having the greatest number of famous scenes, a category in which I include myth, legend, cinema, novel, *manga*, etc.

There are also many famous scenes that are known to all Japanese, but unfamiliar to non-Japanese; very few of them are world-famous.

Dragonball, a Japanese *manga* series written and illustrated by Akira Toriyama, has gained recognition little by little. If this trend continues and images from Japan are accepted more widely, it would provoke a change in the nature of the world. There is no doubt that a change is already emerging if one considers the strong influence of Japanese culture in recent American movies. There is nevertheless a long way to go before it would influence the character of the world.

To return to "Little Snow-White," the primary character associated with madness is the Queen (the stepmother). She had to be the most beautiful woman in the world. Her irrepressible drive to be the best, in the pursuit of which she would use any means necessary, indicates that she has already crossed the second line – madness. Similarly, there is nothing wrong with Olympic athletes going for gold. Rather, their daily efforts to train and discipline themselves are sublime; we see in them one of the noblest states humanity could ever reach. Then, the devil whispers, "Use this drug. It will guarantee you the first prize." As soon as they are tempted by this whisper, they are doomed to madness – doping. Doping gets them into a mess in the real world, like having gold medals taken away, but it gets them into even more trouble psychologically. Noble, daily efforts are suddenly degenerated into serving the devil. God does not give you a drug. The devil, however, concocts them. It is just like a pictorial image of a witch stirring a secret elixir in some mysterious basement. Such a witch's elixir resides in the depths of doping.

I do not know whether the Queen had ever used a secret elixir to get her beauty or not, but she reached madness. When her daughter became seven and turned out to be far more beautiful, the Queen decided to kill her. Here is the scene when the looking-glass answers the Queen, "But more beautiful still is Snow-white."

> Then the Queen was shocked, and turned yellow and green with envy. From that hour, whenever she looked at Snow-white, her heart heaved in her breast, she hated the girl so much.
>
> And envy and pride grew higher and higher in her heart like a weed, so that she had no peace day or night. She called a huntsman, and said: "Take the child away into the forest: I will no longer have her in my sight. Kill her, and bring me back her lung and liver as a token."
>
> (p. 250)

When Snow-white exceeded the evil Queen in "beauty," the Queen was shocked: she became jealous, gnashed her teeth, and hated her daughter. As the jealousy grew like a weed, the Queen probably ranted hysterically that she couldn't bear the sight of her daughter.

So far, so good. This cannot be helped. We often experience these kinds of feelings, if not the ranting. However, the Queen suddenly crossed both the first and second lines: "Bring me back her lung and liver as a token." She did not show so-called psychotic symptoms, but just like the main character of "The Black Cat," her heart stepped into a world that should have been left untrod.

Growing "like a weed" reminds me of the baobab trees in *The Little Prince*. The Queen let the weeds spread. The little prince took good care of the weeds on a day-to-day basis: daily tasks, gathering, attentiveness, and restraint. If he had failed, the possibility of crossing the first line, then the second line – which one should not step over – would have increased.

The Queen could not tolerate the situation of her daughter becoming more beautiful than she. What "beauty" signifies here includes beauty in the common sense of the word, but also the ability to manipulate the human mind, which is one of the devil's attributes. Snow-white exceeded the Queen not only in beauty, but also in magical power. It is equal to the moment when God is no longer God. In the monotheistic world, there is only one God. On the other hand, there is not just one devil, but there is a hierarchy. And the devil also aims at being the one and only God. Perhaps the dynamism of monotheism is being activated behind the numerous doping scandals in the West. There is also a big difference between the gold medal and the silver medal in Japan, but the degree of difference may be unimaginably greater in the West than in Japan. Or in the business world, for instance, the kind of bonus that top executives in major American companies receive is enormous and incommensurate when compared to the salary of top executives in major Japanese companies (though the situation seems to have changed a bit recently). The number one and number two positions are so different from each other.

No woman would not want to be beautiful, but there is going to be big trouble if she realizes her beauty can manipulate the human mind. She then manipulates people around her unawares. Everyone has an innate inclination towards manipulation, but if the response of others to her beauty activates this inclination, everyone becomes trapped. Such a situation gives rise to a fierce conflict in the depths of her mind concerning the pros and cons of controlling this ability to manipulate minds. No one wants to be ugly, but exposing her beautiful face unintentionally manipulates others' minds. "Beauty is very much like a testimonial you cannot reject," is a phrase I read somewhere a long time ago. How challenging not to use such a precious testimonial that has been given to you. What a bothersome conflict to bear! How much energy is consumed by that conflict? The answer is known only to the beautiful, who have become aware of the magical ability to manipulate others' minds. On the other hand, there are always some who want to exercise their magical power to the fullest extent, just like the Queen.

I assume that borderline personality disorder (BPD) is familiar to many people nowadays. It is particularly common in women. Problematic actions, such as wrist-cutting, overdosing, or sexual deviancy are likely to occur in times of stress. Curiously, people with this disorder are often attractive. I have developed the impression that the more beautiful clients are, the more difficult it is to cure them. A positive correlation seems to exist, though not always. The correlation is comprehensible, however, if we think of these dynamics concerning manipulation playing out unconsciously at the core of the clients' pathology. It can also provide a new perspective on BPD that is in service to a deeper understanding.

The Queen's dancing

In the last scene of "Little Snow-White," the crime is revealed and the Queen is brought to justice.

> But iron slippers had already been put upon the fire, and they were brought in with tongs, and set before her. Then she was forced to put on the red-hot shoes, and dance until she dropped down dead.
>
> (p. 258)

Iron, fire, the commons,[6] and death recall the witch trials and the stake. When I visited the torture museum (the Medieval Crime Museum) in Rothenburg, Germany, I felt not only a sense of threat from this terrifying side of human nature, but also an appreciation for the Germans' strong spine in preserving such a museum. The museum allows them to keep reminding themselves that they descended from people who did such horrendous acts. Anyway, it was the world of iron. When a woman was judged to be a witch at the trial, she was given over to fire, the commons, and death. Interestingly, a seeming template for the witch trial had been told long before in folklore. Images, which had been passed on by word of mouth from generation to generation and had taken root in the depths, were perhaps transformed into the reality of torture and the witch trials.

The Queen danced like mad at the very end. She was forced to dance to her death as a punishment. The madwoman at the shrine in my childhood was able to express the "beauty of madness" at least for a moment, although her audience was only me – or perhaps many beyond my knowledge. How about the Queen? There is a large gap between these two women in terms of their quality of soul. The madwoman at the shrine perhaps had schizophrenia. The Queen was less disordered than the madwoman at the shrine in terms of psychopathology, but the disorderedness of her personhood touched the soul. Her pathology reached to the quality of soul, extending beyond the quality of both body and mind. Once this line is crossed, the order of personhood is lost.

The way madness dances in a person's life varies significantly. A scientific giant like Albert Einstein left what are probably unbeatable achievements, as well as an iconic image, over the course of a long history of (likely) maddish thoughts about physics. His accomplishments resulted from the ongoing dance of his maddish thoughts with his ego.

The most difficult piece for the Queen to endure was her beauty no longer being the greatest. Whatever is most unbearable for us has an uncanny way of occurring rather often in our lives. Therefore, it is better not think too much about what would be most unbearable for you. It would more or less increase the likelihood of such things happening. If the Queen had not looked into the looking-glass almost every day, the situation might have been different. She could have manifested her beauty to the fullest, in a manner known only to the Queen. This is the tragedy of bringing objectivity into a place where no objectivity exists. It is important to identify the true nature of this objectivity. The Queen kept asking her question to the looking-glass in an attempt to seek out objective criteria, but this was misguided from the beginning. The looking-glass' answer was nothing but the looking-glass' subjective view. The Queen became overly swayed by the looking-glass' opinion. She was already being taken through the motions.[7] The only way it would be possible for her to shine with her original beauty, in a manner that no one else could ever express, would be to dance actively with the conscious awareness that no objectivity exists.

It is not easy to remain aware that objectivity does not exist. When you realize that no scale can measure things from the outside, the question becomes whether you have your own inner scale. There are times when you must use your own scale, which is less necessary in ordinary times. It takes discipline to develop this inner sense of value. Sliding down to second place was actually a perfect opportunity for the Queen to cultivate her inner sense of value – an affliction from heaven, so to speak. The Queen, however, did not dance to connect her madness with her ego. Her madness departed from her ego, desired the murder of Snow-white, and ordered the huntsman to bring back Snow-white's lung and liver. "The cook had to salt them, and the wicked Queen ate them, and thought she had eaten the lung and liver of Snow-white" (p. 251). The lung and liver were those of a young boar, which the huntsman wittily arranged. It was dreadful nevertheless, since the Queen ate them as Snow-white's. When an affliction from heaven is ignored, people fall into madness very easily.

Remaining grounded

What are we supposed to do to prevent our minds from being overtaken by madness? What should we do to remain grounded? Let me briefly cover this issue here. I will provide greater detail in Chapter 4, but it will only be discussed there from the perspective of therapeutic theory concerning personhood disorders.

The opposite of madness

Let me briefly introduce two figures in the hopes of helping you picture what I mean by madness.

The first figure is a woman who works as a janitor. Whenever I pass her, I find myself looking at her. I sense a distinctive mood that seems all her own. She is entirely absorbed in her task. Her shoulders and arms must become stiff and painful, yet she gives herself up to her work wholeheartedly without any thought of cutting corners. Sometimes I simply feel that she has a genuine attachment to her job, sometimes she looks as if she struggles against something, and sometimes she looks sorrowful. Her mood, as I sense it, is slightly different from moment to moment, but what is always constant is her diligence and pure-mindedness. She lives on the opposite side of what I consider to be madness. Her inviolability is extraordinary, whether she is facing what needs to be done or struggling against something.

The second figure is a man I knew in his thirties. His wife became phobic of men for inevitable reasons. As a result, he could no longer touch her. His wife became afraid of men without exception, and she became terrified of being touched even by her husband. He expressed the pain of not being able to touch his beloved, but he never showed a glimpse of criticism of his wife. "It is not easy, of course," he said with his distinctive smile. His smile was not exaggerated but divine. His stance in the opposite of madness had a great impact on me.

The opposite of the opposite of madness

Many of you know the fairy tale of "The Fisherman and His Wife" from *Grimm's Fairy Tales* (1857/1983). It is an example of the opposite of the opposite of madness, or an example of a person who could not remain grounded.

> There was once upon a time a Fisherman who lived with his wife in a pigsty close by the sea . . . He brought out a large Flounder. Then the Flounder said to him: "Hark, you Fisherman, I pray you, let me live, I am no Flounder really, but an enchanted prince." . . . And with that [the Fisherman] put him back again into the clear water . . . Then the Fisherman got up and went home to his wife in the pigsty.
>
> "Husband," said the woman . . . "Did you not wish for anything first? . . . Go back and call him. Tell him we want to have a little hut" . . . The man still did not quite like to go, but did not like to oppose his wife either, and went to the sea . . .
>
> When the man went home, his wife was no longer in the sty, but instead of it there stood a hut . . . .
>
> (pp. 103–105)

The wife, however, could not remain content with this hut, and she then wanted a stone castle. With each thing granted, her requests escalated more and more – "I must be King" (p. 106), "I will be Emperor" (p. 108), "I will be Pope" (p. 109) – and all came true. And finally the wife said, "I wish to be like unto God" (p. 111). The Fisherman told her request to the Flounder, and the Flounder said, "Go to her, and you will find her back again in the pigsty" (p. 112).

This is the tragedy of someone who could not remain grounded. Nevertheless, she just returned to the original pigsty (and this ending is coherent in all editions), which may seem somewhat mild as an act of God. Nevertheless, it is painful to lose what was once given. The pain of losing treasure that has been given is much greater than not having any treasure at all. Kandata's[8] sorrow (from "The Spider's Thread," a short story written by Ryūnosuke Akutagawa) must have been much deeper after the thread was cut, as was Karoku's[9] after losing his crane wife. Therefore, it is already a severe penalty.

It would have been much better if the wife could have remained somewhere around the stone castle. Yet, once she was caught up in a spiral of greed, she could not help but go all the way.

What would happen if one went all the way in a case involving resentment and bitterness? When the process goes all the way to the bone, it can cause murderous acts. As murder is an act only God can ordain, a man who commits murder can barely remain human. The same applies to those who have experienced almost being murdered. They are forcibly pulled up to the level of God.

What happens if one is murdered? Let's take a look at the world of *Sky-High*.

Poisonous hatred

Sky-High is a Japanese *manga* series (2001; written and illustrated by Tsutomu Takahashi) that was adapted for the screen (2003; directed by Ryuhei Kitamura) as well as a TV drama. In the world of *Sky-High*, people who die as a result of accidents, or who were murdered, go to "the gate of resentment" first. There, a beautiful woman serves as gatekeeper. The gatekeeper presents the dead with three options: to accept death, ascend to heaven, and prepare for reincarnation; to wander around the mortal world as a spirit; or to curse one person in the mortal world to death. If the third option is chosen, however, the chooser is sent to hell with endless suffering and no hope of reincarnation.

The gatekeeper at the gate of resentment recommends the first choice of reincarnation, saying something like, "Why don't you accept your death and wait for your family to come to heaven?" Those who were murdered, however, are too angry to accept her advice. They experience the ultimate conflict of wanting to kill the hateful murderer, yet knowing it will bring them endless suffering. The gatekeeper gives them 12 days to make their final decision, and the dead choose their own way.

There is tremendous anger and resentment at the brink of madness. In *Red Frog*, a Japanese short novel written by Kensaku Shimaki (1946/1969), this is expressed as follows: "Beyond a bad mood, what is called poisonous hatred has thrashed about" (p. 388, our translation). The dead in *Sky-High* suffer from these thoughts of poisonous hatred. The extreme situation depicted by the gate of resentment is an appropriate expression of this dreadful conflict. What is uttered there is barely human. Rather, it is like the words of evil spirits.

Even in clinical practice, there are times when I wonder, "Is this client haunted by something evil?"

In the psychological dynamics occurring between a psychotherapist and client, it is not unusual to feel something so fearsome that it cannot be described with a term like transference. It just strikes with a vengeance. There are times when the psychotherapy must go through a phase almost like a battle between a monster in the client and a monster in the therapist. When a client is too insensitive to the monster inside him or her, and too distant from his or her own ego, the possibility of something drastic happening increases. In such a case, the therapist must be sufficiently sensitive in their stead. Otherwise, the therapist, the client, or people closest to the client may get sick, or in the worst cases, even lose their lives.

Some psychotherapists interpret the occurrence of someone close to the client dying as an inevitable sacrifice for the client's individuation, but sometimes these instances seem to be caused by the insensitivity described above.

The gatekeeper at the gate of resentment – remaining grounded

Let's go back to *Sky-High*. Accepting one's death and departing for heaven must be the best choice based on common sense, but people who suffer at the border of madness cannot easily accept such advice. Such clients are more than aware of which option would be best, yet suffer for not being able to reject the other choices. These clients suffer from their inability to reject. As a result, they remain at the level of resentment, trapped in poisonous hatred. The therapist's words have no power in the face of such a sturdy labyrinth of poisonous hatred.

As poisonous hatred increases, these individuals become restless spirits trapped in the labyrinth or prison of the mortal world. Once this point is reached, they may choose to kill the hated one, thus crossing over even the fear of being sent to hell. They cross over even this eternal agony. This is the true horror of madness.

Now, psychotherapists often play the role of gatekeeper at the gate of resentment, but they are lucky enough to be able to speak with those who suffer from poisonous hatred without specifying an end date – unlike the case of *Sky-High*, which is set at 12 days. But not specifying an end date can also increase the whirling intensity of poisonous hatred even more. The eye of the vortex may then become so sharp and hard that it drills such clients down into even deeper layers of hell as a result. Therefore, 12 days may actually be about right in determining which way to go. There comes a time when what used to be considered poisonous hatred ceases to matter if such individuals force themselves to throw off the poisonous hatred. This can be done by living through wave after wave of poisonous hatred – like a typhoon or an earthquake – and through daily study or work over a long period. Living in the present enables them to leave the past in the past. The past remains in the present if we do not live in the present.

Thus, when a psychotherapist meets clients who are locked up in their own thoughts, it can be very important to empathize with their anguish, while nevertheless requiring them to live in the present and leave the thoughts as they are. The therapist must support clients' efforts to embrace the poisonous hatred or throw it away and make it through the present in one way or another. Of course, psychotherapy can develop in various directions. In some cases, continually listening to their anguish sets clients free. One of my clients, for instance, had been bashing away at her mother for 20 years, and finally became satisfied. Another client had been expressing anguish through rampages for a long time, but when he almost lost his life as a result, the opportunity for a reversal in the situation finally came. No wonder those who care for such individuals have such a tough time supporting them.

Hermann Hesse wrote in "Hell is Surmountable," "You have got to run through the midst of suffering, the midst of despair, to come out to the light again" (1935/2001, our translation). You had better not reject yourself right off the bat for having fallen into the pits of hell. Then, you run through hell as hard as you can so as not to get locked up in it.

When you are deeply hurt, your foundation becomes shaky; it teeters and collapses. What remains after the collapse, however, is true, solid ground. The foundation is tiny, though, so you need to keep spinning like a top not to fall off before a larger foundation is provided.

One day you find that the anguish is no longer as agonizing or bothersome. Furthermore, you gain a treasure that accompanies this bleeding agony. You may find gold when you open up to what you had covered – alchemy.

The types of treasure are infinite in variety. The treasure gained is unique to you, and can even become the core of your personality, as well as the foundation for your subsequent life. It is a unique treasure, which becomes the core of your identity after you are wounded.

It is very important for a psychotherapist to have grit in order to support such people. For one thing, whether or not a psychotherapist can exert this grit at critical moments depends on the psychotherapist's wounds. A psychotherapist needs deep wounds.

In assessment, what is more important than diagnosing the level of psychopathology is not to miss the level of agony. And this is much more difficult than diagnosing the level of psychopathology. Some clients sit in front of a psychotherapist with a nonchalant air, despite being in agony. Listening does not always allow the therapist to grasp the level of agony. The therapist's heart and soul must be able to ascend quite high and to descend deep down into a dark abyss. But this is impossible if the therapist's wounds are shallow. Ascending and descending is only possible through having serious wounds and continuing to struggle against these wounds, or in my terminology, "continuing to dance."

A wound does not always strike us suddenly, nor do we all receive one. But it can be seized with our own hands.

It may sound a bit confusing as an example, but accepting low wages despite deserving high wages could be a wound: it may hurt your pride. If you accept this "negative" aspect in a proactive manner, however, you may find yourself working with a certain zeal that might not appear in simply working for high wages. The janitor has a zeal for her work, and it creates a kind of dignity in her. To put it strongly, I feel a divinity in her. Or the divinity in her comes into play and makes her devoted to mopping this world into cleanliness. Such divinity might be lost in us in the context of high wages.

Divinity exists on a variety of levels. Most likely, its higher levels would not be activated by high wages, while lower levels could be. In terms of the fee for psychotherapy, therapists set a high price once they are qualified, for instance, as Jungian analysts. The price can become several times greater than regular counselors would require. This makes good sense in this world; that is, people with extensive education and qualifications must be paid in keeping with this. But what if the situation is seen from the level of God? The logic of this world would be reversed.

The fee I charge when working as a Jungian analyst is high; otherwise, the work would go amiss. I must admit that I am not at that higher level now. I may not require this same fee if my level goes up. Some considerable degree of discipline and time are necessary to make such a transition.

To add to the issue of wages, there are often times when a low-wage job, such as cleaning or delivering newspapers, serves others' needs more directly. Compared with that, it is doubtful whether a higher-wage job, such as a politician, physician, lawyer, and so on, does as much. It is just one of those things, but it triggers this doubt because such a job involves a research role, engaging in challenging areas where no answer-book is available. High wages are the price paid for the patience to bear the hardship involved with research. Therefore, people in these kinds of professions have a duty to continue studying. A sense of duty should not be the main motivation for a professional, yet it is somewhat necessary. People who are devoted only to research without a sense of duty are easily controlled by the mad scientist archetype. It is just like Dr. Frankenstein, who was so possessed by studying that he created a monster as a result. Considering such a case, it may be better to work with a sense of duty because it keeps a researcher connected to an ethical sensibility. A sense of duty, too, enables one to remain grounded.

Deities (or superhumans) possess power, but do not always exercise their duty.

The mad scientist's tragedy is that of being unable to remain grounded.

Those who remained grounded – Kisuke and Raskolnikov

Some of you may have read *Takasebune,* a Japanese novel written by Ōgai Mori (1916/2006). Here is a synopsis:

Takasebune was a small boat that traveled up and down Takase River in Kyoto, Japan. This boat carried criminals from Kyoto to Osaka who were being sent into exile on a distant island. One day, Shōbei Haneda, an officer in charge of seeing the criminals arrive safely in Osaka, escorted one named Kisuke, who had murdered his younger brother. Shōbei wondered at the looks of Kisuke. "No matter when Shōbei looked at him, Kisuke seemed to be enjoying himself. If Shōbei hadn't been there in the boat with him, he suspected that Kisuke might have begun singing to himself" (p. 11, our translation). Shōbei asked Kisuke what had happened, and found out that he had had quite a life.

Ever since Kisuke had lost his parents as a child, his life was full of struggle. His younger brother could not work due to illness, so the brother tried to commit suicide by slitting his throat. He did not die, however. When Kisuke returned, his brother said, "Forgive me, brother . . . The way things are going, I'll never get my health back. So I thought I might as well end it all. Then you would be free of caring for me" (pp. 29–30).

In the end, Kisuke helped his brother die.

Kisuke, who was sent into exile, said, "Now, thanks to the powers that be, I am being sent into exile. I am being sent off to an island. It seems to me that no matter how bad this island is, it can't be any worse than other places I have lived" (p. 16). Given all the difficulties he went through, Kisuke was content with the prospect of a life without starvation.

> Shōbei began to think about what it meant to be alive in this world of ours. If a person doesn't have enough food to eat, he wishes he were in better health. If he doesn't have any savings, he wishes he did. Human beings are always wishing for what they don't have. They don't know when to stop and say, this is enough. *But then, it suddenly occurred to Shōbei that the person right in front of him, Kisuke, had shown him that people could stop and say, this is enough.*
>
> Shōbei looked down at Kisuke as if he were seeing him for the first time. Kisuke was looking up at the sky. There seemed to be a strange circle of light above his head.
>
> Not taking his eyes off Kisuke, Shōbei called out to him: "Kisuke-san."
>
> (pp. 23–25, emphasis added)

Shōbei addressed Kisuke with *san*[10] upon seeing him remain grounded. We should not stop striving after "a sacred circle of light above the head,"[11] which both the janitor and Kisuke have. Psychotherapists need to be the ones who remain grounded in order to help clients remain grounded. As mentioned previously, the personality structure of people in the state of personhood disorders is disordered due to a pursuit of godhood. The mental attitude of remaining grounded becomes especially important for therapists when seeing clients in the state of personhood disorders.

Let's take a look at Raskolnikov, one of the main characters in *Crime and Punishment*, the novel written by Dostoevsky. Raskolnikov divided people into ordinary and extraordinary, while giving extraordinary men a right to cross over even the law. Considering himself to be extraordinary, Raskolnikov murdered an elderly moneylender. This is the tragedy of one who couldn't remain grounded and who gave himself the rights of godhood. As he became aware that he would not be able to maintain his existence at the level of an extraordinary man, he surrendered himself to justice and accepted his sentence. It was a prostitute, Sonya, who supported him. Although deeply religious, Sonya became a prostitute to help her family. Her deep wound and anguish supported him. It was the kind of help that could only be provided by someone living in hell every day. I do not know if the Judeo-Christian God also placed Himself in hell, but Jesus Christ did bear the cross. This was the root of His salvation.

The disfigured therapist

We live our lives as if trapped by many things. As the Clinical Approach to Life[12] insightfully teaches, we are trapped by lust, money, and greed, whether we are aware of it or not. (The Clinical Approach to Life, which arose in an effort to prevent the recurrence of schizophrenia in Japan, teaches that lust, money, and greed trigger the recurrence of schizophrenia. Yet, it is easy to imagine that they would cause big problems generally.)

The janitor devotes herself to her work, as if she has abandoned all her greed. What she cleans is not only the floor, but also my unclean mind. That is my feeling, at least.

She puts her life into every stroke when she mops. It is not something one can learn superficially, or by simply adopting what appears beneficial.

This lady is my mentor, so to speak. Superficiality does not work in the process of training a psychotherapist. It is quite obvious if one reflects on the fact that undergoing long-term analysis is the most important part of the training to become a Jungian analyst. Whenever I think of her attitude, I am reminded of this basic yet easily forgotten principle.

The role of the gatekeeper at the Gate of Resentment is to allow individuals to let go of revenge. The gatekeeper tries to help them remain grounded. The gatekeeper has to be one who has remained grounded. Just like the janitor, Kisuke, and Raskolnikov (who did not step further into madness, though he murdered), we must remain grounded.

Therefore, it is necessary not to forget, but to remain aware of our own hideous wounds. Everyone is hideously wounded. When we are able to remain grounded as wounded individuals, the disfigured side of therapists is opened up, though it may be far less noble than Sonya.

Disfigured individuals are those who remain aware of this hideous wounding and remain grounded by virtue of it. Such people have a strong will for remaining aware of their deficiencies.

Notes

1 Translators' note: The Chinese character used in writing *jin* means "person," while the one for *kaku* means "rank." *Jin-kaku* can also be translated as "personality."

2 Translators' note: The Chinese character used for *shin* (also pronounced *kami*, depending on usage) means "god."

3 Translators' note: *Mei*: puzzled, *shin*: belief. The closest English word is "superstition," but as is made clear by the definitions later in the paragraph, there are some differences in emphasis. The original Japanese term has been retained to aid in differentiating these.

4 Translators' note: The word "stray" would be a more accurate translation in the context of this passage, but "wanders" is used for consistency in this work.

5 Author's note: What I mean by Christianity here is not the teaching itself of Jesus Christ, but the Christianity which has been acknowledged as legitimate up to today. What we know as the Bible was written from what had been passed down by word of mouth and through the duplication of manuscripts. No original text of the Bible exists.

6 Translators' note: In the English translation of "Little Snow-White," the context in which the stepmother puts on the red-hot shoes is the wedding feast. In the Japanese translation, the term *hiroba* is used, which signifies a public meeting area such as a square, commons, or plaza. This term more readily invites an association to the public commons where witch trials were held.

7 Translators' note: The Queen being "swayed" and "taken through the motions" is meant to contrast with "danc[ing] actively." In other words, the Queen can be passively moved through the dance steps the looking-glass' influence provides for her, or she can proactively engage in her own dance.

8 Translators' note: Written by Ryūnosuke Akutagawa (1892–1927) in 1918. The story depicts a sinner, Kandata, to whom Buddha extended mercy as a result of his one good deed while he was alive: stopping short of killing a spider and thus saving it. Buddha sent down a silvery spider's thread from Paradise to Kandata in Hell. He grabbed hold of it and climbed toward Paradise, but on the way, he looked down and found that other criminals in Hell were following and climbing up the thread. Fearing the thread would break, Kandata yelled at them to back off. At that moment, the thread broke, and Kandata and everyone else fell back into Hell.

9 Translators' note: "The Grateful Crane" (*Tsuru-no-Ongaeshi*) is a Japanese folktale depicting the courtesy returned by a crane to a man named Karoku who saved the crane from a hunter's trap. One day, a beautiful girl visited and wove a roll of gorgeous fabric for him to sell, but forbade him to watch her working.

The fabric was sold at a high price, and as she wove one after another, Karoku soon became wealthy. One day, Karoku could not resist his curiosity, and peeped at her while she was weaving. He saw not the girl, but the battered crane, painfully picking her own feathers and weaving these to make the fabric. The crane soon noticed that she had been seen, felt ashamed, and flew away.

10 Translators' note: *San* means Mr., Mrs., or Ms. in Japanese, and is thus a term of respect.

11 Translators' note: *Gōkō*, which signifies a light emitted from the tuft on the Buddha's forehead. The phrase is in quotation marks to highlight the term, as it is used infrequently in Japanese.

12 Translators' note: *Seikatsu-rinshō. Seikatsu:* life, *rinshō*: clinical approach.

References

Akita, I. (2001). Shinriryōhō-to-ningen: Disfigured hero Shiron [Psychotherapy and human beings: Study on the disfigured hero]. In H. Kawai (Ed.), *Kōza shinriryōhō* [Psychotherapy course] (Vol. 6, pp. 111–153). Tokyo, Japan: Iwanami Shoten.

Akita, I. (2002). Disfigured hero rinshō-hen: Sei-no-itanshatachi [Sexual and gender identity disorders as disfigured hero]. *Bulletin of the Kyoto Bunkyo Center for Clinical Psychology, 4*, 23–28.

Grimm, J. & Grimm, W. (1983). *The complete Grimm's fairy tales*. London, England: Routledge. (Original work published 1857)

Grimm, J. & Grimm, W. (2014). *The complete first edition: The original folk and fairy tales of the brothers Grimm* (J. Zipes, Ed. & Trans.). Princeton, NJ: Princeton University Press. (Original work published 1812)

Hesse, H. (2001). [1935 letter]. In V. Michels (Ed.), *Die hölle ist überwindbar: Krisis und wandlung* (A. Okada, Trans.). Tokyo, Japan: Soshisha. (Original work published 1985)

Jung, C. G. (1989). *Memories, dreams, reflections* (A. Jaffe, Ed., R. Winston & C. Winston, Trans.). New York, NY: Vintage Books. (Original work published 1962)

Mori, O. (2006). *Takasebune* [The Takase boat] (M. Brase, Trans.). Tokyo, Japan: IBC Publishing. (Original work published 1916)

Poe, E. A. (2002). *The complete tales and poems of Edgar Allan Poe*. Edison, NJ: Castle Books. (Original work published 1843)

Saint-Exupéry, A. de (2000). *The little prince and letter to a hostage* (T. V. F. Cuffe, Trans.). London, England: Penguin Books. (Original work published 1943)

Shimaki, K. (1969). Akagaeru [Red frog]. In *Nihon bungaku zenshū* [The complete works of Japanese literature] (Vol. 4, pp. 387–393). Tokyo, Japan: Shueisha. (Original work published 1946)

Takahashi, T. (2001). *Sky-High*. Tokyo, Japan: Shueisha.

Chapter 3

The impossibility of objectivity

As I said in the Preface [Japanese edition],

> There are four characteristics of psycheology. The first is to focus on the *cause of existence* (Akita, 2000). The second is to acknowledge that "objectivity" has no real meaning when dealing with the field of psyche, i.e., objectivity is impossible. The third is to recognize that one's capacity to choose who one really is constitutes the essence of human existence. (p. xvii)

I already mentioned the importance of focusing on the *cause of existence*, mainly in Chapter 1. In Chapter 2, I demonstrated that tragedy occurs when "bringing objectivity into a place where no objectivity exists" (p. 43), and that "the looking-glass' answer was nothing but the looking-glass' subjective view" through the story of "Little Snow-White." In this chapter, I would like to discuss this issue of objectivity and subjectivity more closely. This relates to the perspective from which "we can determine who we are" (p. 5). To recognize the impossibility of objectivity is to thoroughly admit that so-called objectivity is simply meaningless. If we connect that principle to the theory of madness put forth here, we can recognize that objective madness is also impossible. As a result, you can decide for yourself what madness is – and in fact, you should. Putting it strongly, madness does not exist. Only subjective viewpoints on madness exist.

Therefore, the results of mental health evaluations merely reflect the evaluator's subjective view on madness. (This subjective view on madness is the subjectivity of Western mental health, which is inaccurately considered to be highly objective. That is why madness wanders. Again, Western mental health is merely one perspective, and it is neither a universal nor objective gauge.) Western mental health is nothing but subjective reports by clinicians who are not experts on madness, but rather mental disorders.

Physical objectivity does exist. There is a measurable reality with a visible or external scale, such as the number of televisions or grams of an apple.

You do not need an invisible or internal measurement here. You do not need to say, "From an objective point of view, it is . . . ." When the word "objectivity" is used, in contrast, subjectivity comes with it implicitly.[1] That is pretty straightforward.

What about psychology or the mental sphere, then? We tend to pair unconsciously "psychological objectivity" with "psychological subjectivity." That is inaccurate. The validity of objectivity is limited to the physical or material domain. It should not be applied to the psychological or mental domain. Confusion spreads when this point goes unrecognized.

Objectivity exists in mental reality. Anything can exist in one's mental reality, including psychological objectivity.

Psychotherapy begins by accepting the client's unique thoughts and feelings. No matter how unexpected, absurd, unrealistic, or illogical they are, these thoughts and feelings are treated as important in the clinical context. A therapist keeps these thoughts and feelings in mind, though they are obviously odd, as reflections of the client's psychological reality.

Three layers of objectivity

As discussed, there is, first, the world dependent on physical objectivity, which is measurable via external scales, such as five packages, two televisions, or 150 grams. Some philosophical views even cast doubt on this physical objectivity, but in this book I take the position of admitting 150 grams as physically objective.

Second, there is the domain that has some degree of objectivity, although this objectivity is not as accurate. For instance, a score on the college entrance examinations gives you some degree of objectivity. It helps you to see your standing amongst other examinees. You may feel relieved or concerned in knowing this. However, it is not as objective as 150 grams. You may get a high score on Prep Test A, but not as high a score on Prep Test B. Of course, this can happen because the examination questions given and the level of the examinees' ability[2] were different between Prep Test A and Prep Test B. To be bold, the issue is the subjectivity introduced by the writers of Prep Tests A and B. Test Writer A gives questions in Prep Test A, which reflect his or her subjectivity, and the score represents objectivity in the context of this subjective view. No matter how carefully quantified, the class curve is not as objective as 150 grams. This is because the class curve is affected by additional examinee factors, such as their physical condition and their enthusiasm on test day.[3] This level of objectivity should be described in words like "a certain objectivity," "conditional objectivity," or "limited objectivity." It should never be treated in the same manner as the world of 150 grams.

Third, there is a level of objectivity where no objectivity can exist. As I mentioned in the discussion of "Little Snow-White," it is relatively comprehensible that objectivity cannot be applied to beauty. We nevertheless find in the world a reckless will to bring objectivity into this realm. We must pay careful attention to this collective will. This "will" tends to be prompted by earthly desires and greed. When this will is about to come into play, or when objectivity is about to be introduced where no objectivity can exist, greed and earthly desires become intertwined, leading to the emergence of things like beauty contests. The individuals who are selected are certainly beautiful. Their tremendous effort towards that end is respectable, and they may have gained much in the process. They had better not consider their beauty to be objectively proven, however.

Needless to say, the criteria for "beauty" varies widely by region and era. It is hard to imagine that the Miss Universe pageant winner would have won a beauty contest held during the Heian Period[4] in Japan, if such a contest were ever held, or that Ono-no-Komachi[5] would win today's Miss Universe pageant.

Various subjectivities

"In a Grove,"[6] a short story written by Ryūnosuke Akutagawa in 1922, is frequently cited when questions are raised about the nature of facts, truth, or objectivity. This piece belongs to his "dynasty period," and gained inspiration from *Tales of Times Now Past.*[7] "In a Grove" is also known as "the most fictive story among this group" (Yoshida, 1968, p. 217, our translation).

In the story, Masago, a 19-year-old woman of relatively high position, and her husband are attacked by the infamous thug, Tajōmaru, on their way to Wakasa.[8] The husband's body is later found. Tajōmaru, Masago, and her husband's ghost all speak about the incident, but their stories are totally different from one another. The author separates each story by chapter with the following titles: "Tajōmaru's Confession," "The Shrift of a Woman at Kiyomizu Temple,"[9] and "The Dead Husband's Story Told Through a Medium." The existing interpretations of "In a Grove" do not seem to pay attention to the subtle differences of these expressions in the chapter titles: "Confession," "Shrift," and "Story Told Through a Medium."

Tajōmaru's subjectivity

According to Tajōmaru's "confession," he himself was the one who raped Masago and killed her husband.

> Then, the wind lifted the veil, and I saw her face. It was just a glance. The moment after I thought I saw her, I couldn't see her any longer. Maybe that is one of the reasons why I saw her face as a female bodhisattva. In that instant, I decided to steal her by any means necessary, even murdering her husband.
>
> (Akutagawa, 1922/1953, p. 167, our translation)

If the wind hadn't blown then, nothing would have happened. Just like a *Noh* mask,[10] a human face changes in each moment. If the veil had not been lifted at the very moment when her face looked like a female bodhisattva, or someone from another world, nothing would have happened. Because of these two unexpected occurrences, Tajōmaru experienced an attack of madness in that instant. However, the madness was probably not accompanied by so-called psychiatric symptoms in that moment.

According to Yoshida's annotation, a "female bodhisattva" signifies "a Buddha with a female body. The analogy of a beautiful woman is used as no female Buddha really exists" (p. 209). Perhaps deep down, Tajōmaru had become disgusted with himself for continuing to commit acts of theft, murder, and rape. Nevertheless, he could not stop himself from committing them. He might have been begging for something to stop him – it is the same trajectory into madness as "The Black Cat" protagonist stepping over the second line.

Why did she look like a female bodhisattva?

This bodhisattva recalls the dream of Shinran[11] at Rokkakudō Temple.[12] In the case of Shinran, the bodhisattva appeared to him in a dream and said, "I shall be your wife," in order to provide him with lifelong support. In the case of Tajōmaru, the female bodhisattva appeared to him in order to grant the wish lurking in the depths of his mind:

> Suddenly, she clung like crazy onto my arm. As I listened carefully to her fragmented cry, she was saying that either I must die or her husband must die, because having her shame revealed to two men was worse than death. One of us must die, and she would go with whomever was left alive. This is what she gasped out. At that moment, I desperately wanted to kill the man. (Said with somber excitement)
>
> You may say that I am crueler than you. But you will never know until you see her face, especially her burning eyes. When I looked into her eyes, I thought I must have her as my wife, even if it meant being struck by lightning.[13]
>
> (p. 168)

This is just too bizarre. Who would ever cling like crazy onto the arm of the man who raped her? The female bodhisattva (in the form of Masago) would, in order to prevent Tajōmaru from committing another potential crime if he were left alone. Then, Tajōmaru was struck by another madness attack: he desperately wanted to kill the man, and he wanted to have her as his wife even if it meant being struck by lightning. Just as in Shinran's case, Tajōmaru needed this female bodhisattva as his wife – the two must become one flesh.

Tajōmaru released the man, which was uncharacteristic of him, and fought nobly against him. On the 23rd round, Tajōmaru plunged his sword into the man's chest. Tajōmaru looked around, and realized that the woman was gone. Tajōmaru was finally able to demonstrate his heroic side under the female bodhisattva's guidance. In that moment, the female bodhisattva provided Tajōmaru with the mental reality of attaining her as his wife, and then disappeared.

This was all Tajōmaru's "confession," in which he presumably spoke with gratitude of his having been purified. There are various types of confession. For example, a husband confessing to his wife that he ate such and such in the refrigerator yesterday because he was a bit hungry is a confession near the fact. It is rather unnatural to consider Tajōmaru's confession about such an extreme situation as technically accurate and told in a matter-of-fact way. It is impossible to describe what happened with such accuracy as to convince everyone, as it was the kind of story in which the likes of a female bodhisattva appeared. Tajōmaru didn't resist arrest, and requested the ultimate penalty for himself.

The female bodhisattva appeared to Tajōmaru, struggling with his life[14] as he was, and accepted him. Tajōmaru fought heroically as a man, and won. He could then die a victor. Is there any better way for Tajōmaru to die?

A confession is typically given by a person who has done something bad, such as a criminal in a police investigation.

A crime such as murder does not occur in an ordinary state of consciousness. Murder involves either chronic madness or a madness attack. I don't know whether the devil, a bodhisattva, or God appears every time an extreme state is reached, but a client once prefaced his story with, "You wouldn't believe this if I told you." He said this even to me as a therapist, and continued on with a strange story, glancing frequently at me. As soon as the client sensed skepticism or condescension, he stopped talking. "I knew you wouldn't believe me." It is not good to lean in with too much interest, either. It is not unusual to hear odd stories that are wrapped up in too many coincidences, including the appearance of figures that can only be described as gods or bodhisattvas. Such stories are often told, and do not belong to the same dimension as a schizophrenic delusion.

I may have more opportunities to hear to such stories, as I was trained in particular to listen to them. What I mean by training most notably includes a Jungian's training analysis. Part of my practice involves dealing with such magical presentations in the form of dreams.

How much of such a mental reality can be shared in court in front of people who never had such training? As I said before, these things can happen in the mental reality that is crucially important for clients, yet unrealistic.

"I gave up the sword before entering the city. That is it for my confession. Please charge me with capital punishment, as I would hang myself anyway" (p. 169).

Tajōmaru, who wanted to do something to end his life, could finally do so as the one who was embraced by the female bodhisattva, albeit momentarily. Tajōmaru (多襄丸) – what a name, anyway! *Tajō* (多襄) has the same pronunciation as a word meaning "amorous." *Jō* (襄) signifies climbing somewhere high to escape from things like tsunamis that flood towns and villages. It suggests that Tajōmaru might have been amorous, and had characteristics that were easily assailed by tsunamis or flooding. His life may have always been threatened by flooding. Perhaps he was constantly between life and death. If such were the case, rape and murder probably wouldn't mean that much, compared to ordinary people.

The width and depth of the viewer's worldview is always critical in "examining" (*miru*) someone. *Miru*[15] can signify different things: to see (見る), to look (視る), to view (観る), to examine (診る), to nurse (看る), and to conduct [medical] rounds (回る). A clinician must do all this and more in order to examine a client.

Masago's subjectivity

The next story is Masago's. After being raped, she ran to her husband, whose mouth had been stuffed with bamboo leaves to prevent him from speaking.

> Then, I saw an indescribable look in my husband's eyes. As I recall those eyes, I cannot help shivering. He couldn't speak a word, but everything he wanted to say was in his lackluster eyes. It was neither anger nor sorrow reflected there, but a cold light of disdain. Struck more by the color of my husband's eyes than the thug's kicks, I screamed, then fainted.
> (p. 169)

When Masago regained consciousness, she said to her husband, "I cannot be with you any longer. I am prepared to die. However, you must die with me. You have seen me shamed. I cannot let you stay here alive" (p. 169). Masago tried to commit murder-suicide, killing her husband first. She tried to kill herself right after, but couldn't. That is her shrift.

Since ancient times, it is characteristic of Japanese stories for a woman to show anger or disappear once she has been shamed. In the *Kojiki* (*The Record of Ancient Matters*), for instance, Izanami died after giving birth to a fire deity, Kagutsuchi, and became an inhabitant in the underworld. Izanagi, Izanami's husband, missed her so much that he went down to the underworld to take her back. Izanami said, "I will ask the underworld deity, but please don't look at me all the while" (Tsugita, 1977, p. 60, our translation). Izanagi couldn't keep his promise, however, and in looking at his wife, saw her hideously transfigured body. Izanami was humiliated[16] and burned with anger. She sent the Yomotsushikome – monstrous, hideous women of the underworld – to chase Izanagi, but they failed to catch him at the last moment.

There are many more stories with this motif, such as Toyotamahime giving birth in the *Kojiki*, "The Grateful Crane" from Japanese folklore, *The Black Mounds* from *Noh*, and so forth. Should we then take Masago's story of murdering her husband as a straightforward example of the shame motif from ancient times? It seems unlikely. Masago had probably been sensing the cold light of disdain in her husband's eyes for a long time. And this sense became clear in this extreme situation. If it had been an intense but momentary emotion appearing for the first time, generated from the seismic tremor of the husband's heart, she would never have recognized it. But Masago clearly recognized in an instant what she had been faintly sensing. This recognition became an intention to kill him and generated this story of murdering her husband. Masago's heart had already been distant from her husband, but she finally made a decisive break with him in producing this story.

She killed her husband, at least in her mental reality. Regardless of what she had actually gone through, she felt desperately apologetic for murdering her husband. Her apology was deep enough to reach the religious realm. Therefore, the author used the term "shrift" in naming this story.

Tajōmaru's "confession" does not reach the level of a shrift. He did find heroism in concluding his life with the female bodhisattva at his side, but he did not reach deep enough to atone for the numerous crimes he had committed. That's why the author left his story as a "confession."

The husband's (ghost's) subjectivity

Tajōmaru's "confession" and Masago's "shrift" are followed by the story of the ghost of Masago's husband, spoken through a medium. What kind of story did he have to tell even after becoming a ghost? After the thug (Tajōmaru) had his way with Masago physically, he came onto her verbally. Masago seemed to listen attentively to the thug – her husband was convulsed with jealousy.

> "Do you have a mind to be my wife?" . . .
>
> When the thug asked my wife this, she raised her face with a dreamy look. I had never seen my wife look as beautiful as she did then . . . Even

> when I was wandering back and forth between life and death, every time I recalled my wife's reply, I burned with anger. My wife certainly said, "Take me with you wherever you go." (He does not speak for a long while.)
>
> That was not her only sin against me. If that were the only sin, I would not suffer this much. My wife, whose hand lay dreamily in the thug's, was about to go into a grove. Suddenly, she stopped, pale-faced, and turned to point at me under the cedar tree. "Please kill him! I cannot go with you if he is alive." She cried out repeatedly like mad, "Please kill him!"
>
> (p. 170)

Tajōmaru turned to Masago's husband and said, "What do you want me to do with this woman? Kill her or release her? You just nod to reply. Should I kill her?" As soon as she heard this, she ran away. Tajōmaru cut a few ropes tying up the husband, and ran after her. After they were gone, the husband stabbed himself in the chest with the intention to die, and fell into the darkness between life and death.

His desperation must have been beyond imagination: he was tied up by Tajōmaru; witnessed his wife being raped; saw her responding to the thug with a beautiful look, the likes of which she had never shown him; and heard her requesting that he be killed. No wonder he committed suicide and wandered between life and death.

There are many "attacks" in this story. As soon as Masago asked Tajōmaru to kill her husband, Tajōmaru asked him, "What do you want me to do with this woman? . . . Should I kill her?" (p. 170). Such a rapid, attack-like change of mind, however, is appropriate in a way. Tajōmaru behaved properly. Masago's request that Tajōmaru kill her husband also seems too sudden – "pale-faced . . . cr[ying] out repeatedly like mad, 'Please kill him!'" These are madness attacks. But it is also her true, yet hidden, thought – a thought which could only be expressed as an attack.

I wrote, "What kind of story did he have to tell even after becoming a ghost?" But this could be rephrased as "the story that could only be told after becoming a ghost." It is exactly the same as Rokujō-no-Miyasudokoro in *The Tale of Genji*, who became a wraith so she could fully express her resentment and bitterness, which could not have been spoken in human form.[17]

Taken broadly, the true thought that can only be expressed as an attack, and the story that can only be told as a wraith or ghost, are of considerable clinical importance. A clinician must be well aware that these manners of expression do exist.

Masago's husband had always felt jealous of her. I assume this is the case. The feeling had been simmering, but in this extreme situation, it swelled rapidly.

The husband's unconscious generated this story out of the blue.[18] He must have seen Masago's beautiful look many times, but it was simply cast on the retina, without reaching his heart. It was the extremity of this situation that allowed it to finally burst through, reaching his heart with painful intensity.

Shakespeare described jealousy as "the green-eyed monster" (1565/1952, p. 223), but any negative feeling can be a monster, though its eye color may be different. Sometimes negative feelings, in the course of being expressed, become too monstrous for chains to hold. And sometimes negative feelings remain unexpressed, building up in the depths until they explode, as was the case for Masago's husband. The former case can be easily linked to external attacks of violence, while the latter seems related to ghosts or wraiths.

The despair of the small-hearted

You may think such a terrible story doesn't happen too often, but at the level of mental reality, we readily generate such desperate stories. I can say that it is nothing out of the ordinary in clinical practice. It is also typical for there to be big differences between what clients and people around them, such as their family members and partners, report. It is not unusual for individuals to commit suicide, disappear, rampage, shout, or screw up their lives as a result of being locked up in their own story.

Masago's husband experienced this incident as just such a desperate story. Sometimes there is only one truth, and sometimes not. As "In a Grove" depicts so well, the ordinary space-time structure does not exist in such extreme situations. Three independent truths were developing simultaneously.

I cannot see any psychiatric symptoms in these three characters. Tajōmaru was a thug by nature, and was simply struck by one of his attacks. Masago, who had been living her life together with her husband, was probably feeling the cold light in her husband's eyes and trying not to recognize her own true feelings.

Masago's husband was probably small-hearted. His unconscious instantly developed the story out of his desperate delusion and locked him up in it. That is horrifying. Being locked up in one's own thoughts, feelings, and stories is in the nature of what we call madness. These individuals lock themselves up in their own prison.

If we think about this situation commonsensically, it is only the husband who is free from a sense of guilt. Tajōmaru's flagrancy requires no further explanation. While she was in an extreme situation, Masago nevertheless killed her husband, at least in her mental reality. In contrast, her husband was tied up by Tajōmaru, had his mouth stuffed with bamboo leaves, and witnessed his wife being raped. He was merely a victim.[19] It was in this situation, however, that his self-entrapment was symbolically depicted. His small, twisted heart could only see his wife's beauty in such an extreme situation.

Tajōmaru died at the height of selfishness. Masago shrived herself and continued her life, bearing a burden of sin. The most agonized and locked-up one must be Masago's husband. More negative feelings were imposed upon him than he could express as a human being. He was nevertheless the one who generated the most convincing story because of his small-heartedness and sensitivity.[20] His story was the perfect culmination for the novel.

This novel brilliantly depicts how vulnerable objectivity is in the field of psychology. I even feel that this story explains the essence of *Wandering Madness* from the novelist's point of view.

Human beings need a certain level of mental or psychological safety. We all want a foundation. Sometimes parents' influence suffices as the foundation, and other times communal conventions do, such as those found in religions.

In our time, parental influence, communal conventions, and religious influence have wavered. Where should we seek the mental or psychological standard, then? This issue also has something to do with the current dependence on psychiatric medicine. All in all, wandering without a home is hard. Presumably, the increased number of people diagnosed with borderline personality disorder (BPD) follows from this trend.

People with BPD don't have a foundation. As the following chapter's subtitle indicates, we are all borderline to a greater or lesser extent, and are at the borderline. No one's foundation is as solid as they think. The next chapter will discuss issues associated with BPD, which represents the human condition so well.

Notes

1 Translators' note: i.e., as soon as there is any reference made to the objectivity of something, there is a (potentially implicit) contrast being made to subjectivity.
2 Translators' note: The Japanese college entrance exams use scaled scoring. Thus, a given examinee's score will be influenced by the performance of everyone else in the group.
3 Translators' note: In Japan, all students take formal examinations, such as the college entrance exam, on the same day.
4 Translators' note: 794–1185.
5 Translators' note: A poet of the early Heian Period (ninth century) known as one of the most beautiful women of all time in Japan. Her elegiac poetry concerned the passionate feeling of love.
6 Translators' note: *Yabu-no-naka*. Made internationally famous by Akira Kurosawa's cinematic adaptation of it in *Rashōmon* (Daiei Motion Picture Company & Kurosawa, 1950).
7 Translators' note: *Konjaku Monogatari*. A collection of stories written and edited during the late Heian Period (794–1185), the authors and editor of which are unknown.

8 Translators' note: In Fukui Prefecture on the main island of Honshu, Japan.
9 Translators' note: In Kyoto, Japan.
10 Translators' note: *Noh* is a highly refined and stylized form of Japanese theater in which many characters wear wooden masks crafted by artisans. The masks are designed to reflect different expressions depending on the angle at which they are viewed. Even when actors are not wearing wooden masks, their faces are considered to be masks themselves (*hitamen*).
11 Translators' note: 1173–1262. Japanese Buddhist monk who founded the True Pure Land sect (*Jōdo Shinshū*). In early Japanese Buddhism, when monks were strictly prohibited to marry, Shinran was the first to have a wife. He had a revelatory dream of a bodhisattva permitting a monk to marry a woman, as the bodhisattva would incarnate herself as his wife.
12 Translators' note: In Kyoto, Japan.
13 Translators' note: *Kaminari* ("thunder"), which literally means "*kami*'s rumbling," was believed to be a manifestation of *kami* ("god") in ancient times. The implication here is that Tajōmaru wanted Masago even if it would incur the wrath of the *kami* and bring him death in the next instant. "Lightning" is used here instead of the more literal "thunder" to make use of the phrase "struck by lightning."
14 Translators' note: Tajōmaru probably felt burdened by all of his previous crimes and did not know what to do with himself. He had become sufficiently desperate in his attempt to "come clean" that he was likely thinking about death as a potential solution.
15 Translators' note: The Japanese language has many homonyms, such that a single spoken word signifies multiple words in written form. The author is making the point that these written words, which have distinct meanings at the surface, nevertheless bear a notable similarity at a deeper level.
16 Translators' note: In ancient Japan, death was abhorred as something unclean. Because purity and brightness were of paramount importance, it was very shameful for Izanami to be seen in her deathly, unclean form by her husband.
17 Translators' note: *The Tale of Genji* (*Genji Monogatari*), written by Murasaki Shikibu during her time as a lady-in-waiting in the middle of the Heian Period (794–1185). The story portrays the life and romances of Prince Genji, depicting the medieval court life of Japan. It is generally considered the first novel ever written.

Rokujō-no-Miyasudokoro, the widowed empress, was one of Genji's mistresses. However, Genji became reluctant to see her because of her nobleness and keen intellect. Though she loved Genji deeply, Rokujō repressed her feelings of true love because she considered expressing them to be inappropriate of her age and high status. When Genji married another woman, her jealousy transformed her into an evil spirit that haunted Genji's wife.
18 Translators' note: The Japanese equivalent of this idiom is "out of a grove," suggesting an association with the title of the story being referenced: "In a Grove."
19 Translators' note: Masago is physically abused in being raped and is the primary victim in this respect. However, her psychological perspective or resilience is such that she does not remain as narrowly defined by the event as does her husband.
20 Translators' note: The husband's story is the most convincing because he is the most locked up in it. Having the least tolerance for any outside perspective (his sensitivity), he believes his story entirely, and is thus the most convincing in relating it to others.

References

Akutagawa, R. (1953). Yabunonaka [In a grove]. In *Akutagawa Ryūnosuke shu: Gendai Nihon bungaku zenshū* [A collection of Ryūnosuke Akutagawa stories: The complete works of Japanese contemporary literature] (Vol. 26, pp. 166–170). Tokyo, Japan: Chikuma Shobo. (Original work published in 1922).

Daiei Motion Picture Company (Producer) & Kurosawa, A. (Director) (1950). *Rashômon* [Motion picture]. Japan: Daiei Tokyo Studios.

Shakespeare, W. (1952). Othello, the Moor of Venice. In R. M. Hutchins (Series Ed.), *Great books of the western world* (Vol. 27, pp. 205–243). Chicago, IL: Encyclopædia Britannica. (Original work published 1565)

Tsugita, M. (1977). *Kojiki: Zenyakuchū* [Kojiki, with complete annotations] (Vol. 1). Tokyo, Japan: Kodansha Gakujyutsu Bunko.

Yoshida, S. (1968). Kaisetsu [Interpretation]. In R. Akutagawa (Ed.), *Jigokuhen* [Hell screen]/*Chūtō* [The robbers]. Tokyo, Japan: Shinchobunko.

Chapter 4

The departure from godhood

Everyone is borderline and at the borderline

This book introduces the perspective of *psycheology* and develops it while raising questions concerning existence and madness. In this chapter, I proceed further, focusing on personhood disorders,[1] especially borderline personality disorder (BPD).

Mental disorders are sometimes categorized into levels of psychopathology: normal, neurotic, personhood disordered, and psychotic. The difference between neurosis and psychosis was a notable topic of debate until a few decades ago. This debate, however, has not actually concluded. I was recently asked to write an article about the issue of "neurosis versus psychosis" in an encyclopedia of clinical psychology (Akita, 2011). In that article, I discuss how "normal" and "personhood disorder" can be productively compared, just as "neurosis" and "psychosis" are.

So-called normal people often skip over the neurotic state into the state of personhood disorder. In addition, people in a state of personhood disorder sometimes suddenly return to the normal state without passing through the neurotic state in the course of treatment. This bypass does not always occur, however. While the mental health perspective suffices for the "neurosis versus psychosis" dynamic in most cases, the perspective of *psycheology* becomes necessary for the "normal versus personhood disorder" dynamic. It is essential to reconsider the meaning of human existence and madness beyond the realm of the mental health perspective.

As mentioned in the Preface [Japanese edition], this chapter discusses therapeutic theory, and as a result, the tone of this chapter may sound a bit different from the rest of the book.

The English term "personality disorder" was first translated as *jinkaku-shōgai*[2] by The Japanese Society of Psychiatry and Neurology. This translation was used in the Japanese version of DSM-IV (1995), but was modified to *personality-shōgai* in DSM-IV-TR (2002). In the ICD nomenclature, it was translated as *jinkaku-ijyō* ("abnormality of personhood") in the ninth edition (as cited in Ootsuki, 1978), and *jinkaku-shōgai* in the 10th edition (1993). *Seikaku-shōgai* ("characteristics disorder") is another Japanese term used as a translation of personality disorder. All of these are Japanese words for the English term personality disorder, and there is no consensus as of yet for using a single term in Japanese.

It is okay to be multifaceted

As you see, there are some variations when translating "personality disorder" into Japanese, which has advantages and disadvantages. *Jinkaku-shōgai* (personhood disorder) was the most popular translation until recently, but *personality-shōgai* (personality disorder) is becoming more mainstream. *Seikaku-shōgai* (characteristics disorder) does not stand much of a chance, but I am not in favor of abandoning it completely.

In my opinion, personality disorder does not have to be standardized into one translated term. We just have to use the most appropriate term for the situation in each clinical context. Terms such as "pseudoneurotic schizophrenia," "multiple personality disorder," and "monomania" are no longer used in today's clinical practice, but they don't need to be relinquished for that reason alone. When the word "psychopathy" was banned, Schneider said, "the word 'psychopathy' is dying, but the psychopath lives on" (as cited in Nishiyama, 2004, p. 138, our translation). That is true. Clinical conditions that can only be described in certain words and concepts definitely exist.

Behind each concept lies a unique interpretation of the world. Preserving various concepts means retaining diversity in how we interpret the world. Therefore, it would probably be ideal to say that it is "better" to be multifaceted, rather than that it is "okay" to be multifaceted. While we should continue to seek more appropriate concepts, we should not so readily abandon a cosmology or interpretation of the world.

The state of disordered personhood

In this book, I primarily use the term *jinkaku-shōgai* (personhood disorder) to indicate the English term personality disorder. I also try to add "state" to this term whenever possible: the disordered personhood state or the state of disordered personhood.

First of all, I would like to explain why I chose the word *jinkaku* (personhood) over other terms to describe personality.

As part of my clinical stance, I incorporate the perspective of *tamashii* (魂; "soul" or "mana"), for which terms like "characteristics" or "personality" seem too mild. As shown in Figure 4.1, I see *jinkaku* (personhood) as

Personality (*persona* or *hitogara*: "personality pattern")

↓↑

Personhood (*jinkaku*: "mastery of being oneself")

↓↑

Soul (魂, *tamashii*: "soul, mana")

Figure 4.1

being located between personality at the surface layer and *tamashii* (soul, mana) at the deeper layer. Personality is derived from the Latin word *persona* ("mask"), so it carries the meaning of the face one shows to the outer world. Therefore, it may be more appropriate to consider it as the side one shows to society, rather than simply a surface layer. Or *hitogara*[3] ("personality pattern") could be a better word. *Hitogara* emphasizes the impression on others, and actually there are some cases in which *hitogara-shōgai* ("personality pattern disorder") seems to be the most appropriate translation for personality disorder.

I do not mean to cling to the word *jinkaku* (personhood). In clinical practice, whenever sharing the diagnosis with a client is necessary, I endeavor to use the word most likely to increase the possibility of therapeutic success. Personally, I find the word *jinkaku* (personhood) to be a good fit in many cases; but this is only my personal impression, so it should not just be applied directly to clinical practice.

Next, the reason I add the word "state" to "personhood disorder" is because disordered personhood is not something fixed. With borderline cases that begin in adolescence, for instance, the diagnostic criteria are often not met after the age of 40. Nevertheless, clients themselves will often be incredibly certain that their inability to function is a result of problems associated with personality characteristics that cannot be changed. Therapists themselves sometimes believe this to be the case. We must be well aware that it is a state.

The reason why individuals exhibiting borderline features who are above age 40 sometimes do not meet the diagnostic criteria is due to the traditional therapeutic method.[4] Taking so much time for the treatment is intolerable. The duration of therapy would be much reduced if we focused most of the attention on clients' acting out. Except in severe cases, it is not unusual for therapy to end within three to five years.

The mastery of being human

The Chinese characters used for *jinkaku* (personhood) are 人格 (人: *jin;*[5] 格: *kaku*). The original meaning of 格 is "to master." Therefore, the subtext of the word *jinkaku* is that human beings must follow and master the way of being themselves. However, as mentioned in the previous chapter, many of those who have personhood disorders often wish for godhood (*shinkaku*),[6] which gets them off the track of being themselves.

The state of being disordered

If *jinkaku-shōgai* (personhood disorder) indicates a dysfunctional state in being human, then what kind of conceptualization underlies the English term personality disorder? If *jinkaku-shōgai* (personhood disorder) were merely considered as the translated Japanese term for personality disorder, we wouldn't need to discuss the difference between them. However, that is not right. The terms are obviously different.

As another example, "psychotherapy" is translated as *shinri-ryōhō* in Japanese (*shinri*: psychology; *ryōhō*: therapy), but psychotherapy and *shinri-ryōhō* do not mean the same thing. The idea that the original term and the translated one are identical is wrong. They have different connotations. A word is a mode of expression loaded with a whole cosmology. We must be sensitive to the difference between words. The translated word tends to be identified with the original word overly much. It may be one of our diseases. What about a "camera" and *shashinki* (*shashin*: picture, photo; *ki*: machine)? These words indicate entirely, or almost entirely, the same object. The original term and its translated term have little or no difference when they refer to something concrete or physical. When it comes to concepts, however, there is a difference.

"Dis-order" means a state of dysfunction in the order of things. What order? The divine order. The diagnostic criteria of mental illness in the West originated primarily in Germany and were derived from the Christian tradition. In the West, the Christian God underpins many things, even if that is not verbalized. It is same in psychiatric diagnosis. To secede from the providence of God is disorder.

If "the providence of God" is rephrased to "order as God's ordinance," an attitude that challenges the order is disordering. In Christianity, godhood must be pursued; individuals must approach God as much as possible. In order to do so, they should pray and live humbly. At the same time, they must not step over the absolute boundary between human and God. Stepping over the border is disorder. Those called saints have stepped over, but they have a heightened awareness that they are not God.

In Japan, there is a mild continuity between humans and gods. Once a person dies, the soul remains in a mountain behind the home, and occasionally returns. In the meantime, this soul becomes a god. In a Japanese village, humans and gods blend, flowing together in the cosmic river.

While the conception of the divine differs in the East and West, the deep pathology that gives rise to disordered personhood in the pursuit of godhood is shared. But again, what constitutes the divine and how humans relate to it are quite different between East and West, so I expect you to take this commonality as the essential or distilled form of explanation about this deep pathology.

Awareness of being bad

When certain individuals diagnose and begin treating other individuals with mental disorders, they must remember not to place themselves on the "normal" side. Everyone is bad, without much difference.

Some sufferers run to a *Yakuza* boss for help. Spending some time with a boss who is aware of his or her badness may help them to live through that moment. Some may run to a Buddhist monk. If the monk is someone who laments, as the youngest disciple, his or her inability even to approach Buddha, yet continues the discipline, the sufferers may feel eased a bit. The same happens in Christian churches.

One of my friends visited me the other day. We got on the topic of everyone being bad. My friend said that we are all bad because "we can only continue our lives by killing others." I said, "But what about vegetables, fruit, or fish? They look as if they don't care whether they are killed." "Not vegetables and fish," he said, "but fruit certainly looks as if it wants to be eaten." At a later date, I told this story to another friend, who said, "I don't think fruit looks like that."

If we see things from this perspective, we realize how harmful we are to other beings in the pursuit of our survival. I asked a Christian and a Buddhist about their perspectives on this issue. From the Christian perspective, fish and meat are created to be eaten by human beings, so there is no issue in eating them; while from the Buddhist perspective, human beings are created as they are, so there is no issue in eating fish and meat if it is done with gratitude. No matter how much gratitude we feel in eating, however, the fact of killing living things will not relieve the guilt of surviving by killing other living things.

Yet, we all need to eat in order to live on; therefore, we must at least be aware of our badness and the great burden this entails.

Fellow sufferers commiserate

When I work as a psychiatrist or psychotherapist, clients visit my office one after another. There surely exist some cases where clients are best examined from the diagnostic perspective. Yet, the diagnosis is given only because the client is viewed from such a diagnostic perspective. Since many diagnoses already exist these days, clients are often examined based on these diagnoses.

However, if I engage with clients while recognizing that I am someone of little consequence, as a sinner or a bad person, the situation becomes very different. The attitude in diagnosing becomes more like that between fellow sufferers commiserating.

Such an attitude in the therapist can serve as a foundation for turning the client's projective identification (or *participation mystique*, in Jungian terms) – a common mental mechanism in people with BPD – into something therapeutically beneficial. This attitude can become a container. Therefore, it is necessary for a psychiatrist or psychotherapist to have the attitude of being a fellow sufferer from the beginning. Then, we meet clients as experts in "disease." Being an expert in disease also means being deeply aware of our own diseased nature.

A former client kept bad-mouthing (her husband) for 20 years. Meeting such a client repeatedly is not an easy thing to do for psychotherapists who lack awareness of their own badness. Otherwise, I would say, "That's enough!" When I reflect on myself, however, I can find many things about which I almost say to myself, "That's enough," as well. If therapists keep this in mind while seeing clients, the therapy proceeds differently.

A self-help group can be very effective, such as for people who are dependent on alcohol or drugs. They support each other in groups like Alcoholics Anonymous. In terms of cases involving only alcohol dependency, it is said that nothing is known to be as therapeutic as support groups like Alcoholics Anonymous. This reminds me of how important it is to foster the attitude of fellow sufferers supporting each other.

We do not suffer as much, compared to our clients. For this reason, we must keep our own disorderedness firmly in mind. A therapy case is unlikely to proceed as smoothly without this awareness; the more severe the client, the more difficult the progress if a psychotherapist is not aware of his or her own disorderedness.

A mind that never disrespects others

Not disrespecting clients is easier said than done. Psychiatrists are so busy that they tend to treat clients roughly. And it is not rare to go well beyond this, like looking down on clients or saying something derogatory to them. I have heard secondhand that a psychiatrist will sometimes say, "We cannot see someone like you."

Seeing clients with a personhood disorder requires a lot of energy from therapists. Not a few psychiatrists may think, "I wish the client would not come back." Some psychiatrists see a client only monthly, though weekly would be more appropriate (because it is exhausting). The situation would be different if they maintained awareness of their being sinners or bad people, and they could commiserate as fellow sufferers. Needless to say, this is about therapists' attitudes, and it is another question altogether whether their discussing their own badness with clients would be therapeutic or not. Sometimes it can be effective, and sometimes it brings stagnation or even deterioration in the therapy.

1. The history of personhood disorders

Where did the concept of personhood disorder originate?

There are many odd people in this world. Among them are some who cannot be categorized as psychotic. They are not psychotic, but very odd. How should we refer to them? This is where the concept of what are now called personhood disorders emerged.

Insanity without delusion

It is difficult to locate the starting point for the concept of personhood disorders. It is common to set it around the age of Philippe Pinel, a psychiatrist famed for releasing the mentally ill from chains – literally. If I had to name only one famous person in the field of Western psychiatry, it would be Emil Kraepelin, but perhaps Pinel would be second. Pinel introduced the concept of "insanity without delusion" in 1801. He pointed out that there was a cluster of people who did not seem ordinary, but were not psychotic, either.

Monomania

Jean-Étienne Dominique Esquirol was a pupil of Pinel, and proposed the concept of "monomania." People with monomania acted and behaved quite normally except in one particular area. It might be a fire-setting habit, a tendency to wander off, or an inclination towards thievery. People with such habits did set fires, wander off, and steal, but they were quite normal except for their one habit. Pinel found that such a cluster certainly existed, and named it monomania. Pinel and Esquirol were both French.

Moral insanity syndrome

In the United Kingdom, James Cowles Prichard proposed the concept of "moral insanity syndrome" in 1835. As the name implies, it was a condition in which individuals acted in a manner considered insane to the moral sensibilities, without any hesitation, yet showed no symptoms of psychosis.

Degeneration theory

Back to France. Most importantly, Benedict Morel introduced "degeneration theory" in 1857. According to the theory, the model for human beings was Adam, and they were originally perfect in the condition of Adam. In the wake of Adam's sin, however, he was negatively impacted by the outer world. As a result, the "degenerate" appeared. That is what this theory was about.

According to the theory, a person affected by this degeneration became somewhat neurotic. The next generation would suffer neurosis itself, the one after that psychosis, followed by dementia, and finally death. What a frightening explanation. It spread throughout Europe in the late 19th century, especially in the 1880s.

Morel's teacher was Jean Pierre Falret, who offered the concept of "circular insanity" – Kraepelin incorporated it into the concept of "manic depression." Falret's teacher was Esquirol. Esquirol's teacher was Pinel. As one can see from the lineage, Morel was quite mainstream in the psychiatric field. Such traditional psychiatrists would have said that an illness developed because Adam committed the original sin.[7]

Superior degeneration

Another psychiatrist who followed Morel's theory was Valentin Magnan. He delivered the theory of "superior degeneration." While Morel found the ideal model in Adam, Magnan thought that human beings could develop despite the Fall, such that the ideal model lay in the future. And he thought there were people who deserved to be called "superior degenerates"[8] among the degenerates. I take this to be one of the ancestral concepts of the *disfigured hero* (Akita, 2001).

Anyway, the latter part of the 19th century was the most important period in terms of establishing psychiatric medicine, and it was Morel's theory that spread and had enormous influence throughout Europe during this time. Lombroso from Italy, for instance, was known for his study of geniuses and criminals, and at the root of his study was the theory of degeneration. As another example, Krafft-Ebing from Austria developed the concept of "*psychopathia sexualis*," the root of which was the theory of degeneration as well.

The psychopath

Julius Ludwig August Koch of Germany developed the concept of "psychopathic inferiority" (1891). It was around this time that the idea of the psychopath began to take root.

Subsequently, Kraepelin began using the term "psychopathic personality" (1910s). He divided psychopathic personality into the following seven subgroups: excitable, unstable, impulsive, eccentric, lying and swindling, antisocial, and quarrelsome. His proposal followed Koch's by a few decades.

Both Koch and Kraepelin saw the psychopath as occupying a position in between normal and psychotic, and thus might be termed middle theorists.

In the 1920s, Kurt Schneider, a pupil of Kraepelin, proposed 10 subcategories, which became the basis for the theory of personality disorders today: hyperthymic, depressive, insecure, fanatical, self-seeking, emotionally unstable, explosive, affectless, weak-willed, and asthenic. These are presumably self-explanatory to a sufficient degree that you can grasp more or less what each subcategory was intended to signify.[9] Schneider saw the psychopath as an independent concept (from what are now called personality disorders), not as something in between normal and psychotic. He insisted that there was an independent unit that could be called psychopathic.

Around the same time, Ernst Kretschmer published *Physique and Character* (1921).[10] He was a middle theorist. His idea, which emphasized continuity, was that when the temperament worsened, it would turn into a "pathologic temperament," then become a "disorder" in more severe cases.

Taking Schneider's typology as the foundation, to which Millon later contributed, this entire stream poured into the *Diagnostic and Statistical Manual of Mental Disorders* (DSM).

The multiaxial diagnostic system of the DSM[11]

The First Edition of the DSM was published in 1952 and the Second Edition in 1968. It was the Third Edition (1980) that significantly changed the world of mental health, as it presented the "multiaxial evaluation" (p. 23) for the first time: Axis I for "Clinical Syndromes," Axis II for "Personality Disorders," Axis III for "Physical Disorders and Conditions," Axis IV for "Severity of Psychosocial Stressors," and Axis V for "Highest Level of Adaptive Functioning Past Year." Before DSM-III, mental conditions were considered continuous: normal, to neurotic, then to personality disorders, and finally to psychosis. Since the multiaxial diagnostic system of DSM-III was introduced, however, personality disorders have been excluded from this continuity.

That is, neuroses (anxiety disorder), bipolar disorder (mood disorder), and schizophrenia are categorized on Axis I. The system requires that personality disorders be assessed separately, on another dimension. Thus, a clinician must examine a client at two different levels. This stance is neither that of middle theorists like Koch and Kraepelin, who considered personality disorders to exist along the continuum with other mental disorders, nor that of Schneider, who did not suppose either continuity or another dimension. This approach was continued in DSM-III-R (1987), DSM-IV (1994), and DSM-IV-TR (2000).

Personality disorders

DSM-IV-TR divides personality disorders into three groups. (The following summary is based on the work of Dr. Naoki Hayashi, 2005.)

Cluster A – The "odd, eccentric" cluster

Paranoid personality disorder

This disorder is characterized by a pervasive distrust and suspicion of others. Such individuals insist they are right and create discord with others. Their cognition and judgment are self-centered and narrow. (People with paranoid personality disorder are likely to develop delusional disorder and schizophrenia, paranoid type. This disorder tends to be found more frequently in men.)

Schizoid personality disorder

People with this disorder seem aloof and cold. They are antisocial, isolated, and lack interest in others. (Schizoid personality disorder was once considered the premorbid personality of someone who came to have schizophrenia. It tends to be found more frequently in men.)

Schizotypal personality disorder

This disorder first appeared in DSM-III. (In ICD-10, it is treated as a subtype of schizophrenia, not as a personality disorder.) The conversation of such individuals is eccentric with poor content. Their clothes and behaviors are often odd. Their thoughts are ambiguous and overly abstract. Their emotional expression is restricted in its range and often inappropriate. They are isolated from relationships. They sometimes talk to themselves, and develop strong beliefs in their intuition. (People with schizotypal personality disorder are likely to develop schizophrenia.)

Cluster B – The "dramatic, emotional, erratic" cluster

Borderline personality disorder

This disorder corresponds to emotionally unstable personality disorder in ICD-10. People with this disorder tend to experience unstable emotions and interpersonal relationships. They have an intense anxiety about being abandoned, and show impulsive behaviors that expose them to danger, including self-injury, suicide attempts (such as wrist-cutting or overdosing), and overspending. Their identity is diffuse. Psychosis-like symptoms, including paranoid and dissociative reactions, as well as idealizing and devaluing others, also distinguish this disorder. (BPD is more likely to co-occur with many other mental disorders, such as major depressive disorder. People with this disorder are seen at high rates in clinical practice. This disorder tends to be found more frequently in women.)

Narcissistic personality disorder

People with this disorder are arrogant and grandiose. They need attention and admiration from others, and cling to their reputation. They believe in their superiority. They may over-idealize others. People with narcissistic personality disorder become depressive and intensely angry when others criticize them or show a lack of interest in them. People with this disorder have little compassion for others. (Narcissistic personality disorder is more likely to co-occur with major depressive disorder and dependency on alcohol and drugs. This disorder tends to be found more frequently in men.)

Antisocial personality disorder

People with antisocial personality disorder engage in antisocial, violent behaviors that disregard and violate the rights of others. They are impulsive and irresponsible with little sense of guilt. It is this group that is the closest equivalent to the term psychopath. People with this disorder are insensitive to the feelings of others, showing no empathy. They are rarely trustworthy or honest. (Antisocial personality disorder is more likely to co-occur with dependency on alcohol and drugs. This disorder tends to be found more frequently in men.)

Histrionic personality disorder

People with histrionic personality disorder attempt to capture the attention and interest of others. Their appearance and behaviors are flamboyant and theatrical. Their expressions of emotion are exaggerated and superficial with little authenticity. People with this disorder are highly suggestible and easily influenced by others. (This disorder is found predominantly in women.)

Cluster C – The "anxious, fearful" cluster

Dependent personality disorder

People with dependent personality disorder tend to be overly dependent on others. They always need others' advice and instruction for their own behaviors and decisions. They are compliant and do not take responsibility. People with this disorder feel impotent and lonely when not supported by others. (Dependent personality disorder is more likely to co-occur with major depressive disorder and panic disorder, with or without agoraphobia. This disorder tends to be found more frequently in women.)

Obsessive-compulsive personality disorder

People with this disorder give the impression of being stubborn, inflexible, and highly organized. They cling to orderliness. This disorder is characterized by perfectionism, over-conscientiousness, logical thinking, and a narrow spectrum of feelings without warmth. They are indecisive in an attempt to avoid intense feelings or something unknown. (Obsessive-compulsive personality disorder tends to be found more frequently in men.)

Avoidant personality disorder

People with avoidant personality disorder are afraid of failure, reluctant to engage interpersonally, and likely to be withdrawn. They avoid situations where they may be rejected, or that might involve intense stimuli. People with this disorder experience anxiety and nervousness due to feeling uncertain and inferior. (Avoidant personality disorder often co-occurs with social phobia.)

That is how personality disorders are categorized. If you reflect on yourself, you may find some overlapping features between your personality and these personality disorders. These categorizations look well organized, but are troublesome when used in clinical practice. Many cases fall in a gray area – for instance, someone who appears borderline but is more or less narcissistic and antisocial.

The preface of DSM-IV-TR explains that "no substantive changes in the criteria sets were considered, nor were any proposals entertained for new disorders, new subtypes, or changes in the status of the DSM-IV appendix categories" (2000, p. xxix), giving the impression that this categorization was so complete that it did not require any further revision. Yet the categorization is questionable.

Dr. Takashi Okada proposed the concept of "grandiose self syndrome" (2005). Through many cases he had observed at a juvenile detention and juvenile classification home,[12] he wrote that there were individuals who certainly had problems at the level of personality disorders, yet didn't meet any criteria. If the term grandiose self syndrome were used, the situation could be well depicted, he said. I found his idea very encouraging because it appears to be close to my perspective, which sees the fundamental pathology of personhood disorders as seeking godhood unconsciously.

Among the various personality disorders described above, BPD is the one most commonly encountered in clinical practice. Now, therefore, I will focus my discussion on this disorder.

Borderline personality disorder

In discussing the history of personhood disorders, there is another stream worth considering – the study of the borderline case.

The history of the borderline case

In 1953, Robert Knight introduced the concept of the "borderline state," which was rooted in clinical practice. Around the same time, Melitta Schmiedeberg, a daughter of Melanie Klein, proposed a similar concept.

If we trace back even further, Wilhelm Reich and Franz Alexander introduced the concepts of the "impulsive character" and the "neurotic character" when Schneider and Kretschmer were active. In 1934, Helene Deutsch proposed the "'as-if' personality," which became one of the precursors in the study of the borderline case. In the 1940s, Paul Hoch and Phillip Polatin introduced "pseudoneurotic schizophrenia." It was a breakthrough concept, as it found a cluster that became even worse when treated as a neurosis. This cluster showed pervasive anxiety and a wide variety of neurotic symptoms. Around the same time, Gregory Zilboorg introduced "ambulatory schizophrenia." Both pseudoneurotic schizophrenia and ambulatory schizophrenia were basically considered to be schizophrenia (although Knight saw the borderline case as an intermediate state between neurosis and psychosis).

In the 1960s and 1970s, Otto Kernberg and Justin Masterson started to play an active role. Kernberg introduced the concept of "borderline personality organization." He distinguished borderline personality organization from neurotic personality organization and psychotic personality organization, and emphasized splitting and projective identification as the basic pathology of the borderline case. Masterson, on the other hand, took particular note of "abandonment anxiety," and considered acting out as a defense against abandonment anxiety. Once acting out was restricted and the defense collapsed, anxious and depressive symptomatology, the treatment of which was primary to the improvement of such clients, would begin to appear. A critical situation would then follow. Masterson said overcoming this crisis was important. He also examined the borderline case in relation to depressive disorders. While Kernberg emphasized an innate factor, Masterson stressed an attitude resembling the mother's in child-rearing, and even remarked on the importance of the therapist's maternal caring in the therapy.

Acting out

Many therapists, including Masterson, have pointed out the importance of limit setting for acting out.

As mentioned, Masterson thought that the restriction of acting out would be so challenging for clients that a crucial psychotherapeutic stage would begin from there. Yet, this is not always the case, at least from my own clinical experiences in Japan. There are far more clients in the borderline state who feel better after they are prevented from acting out.

This issue is delicate and important, so that it needs to be considered more thoroughly.

Constructing the levee

First, I would like to explain how I see the borderline case.

Streetscape

Imagine the mind of borderline clients as a streetscape. There are various houses, stores, and parks in the town. I perceive that the streetscape of the borderline case is of fine quality. It is even attractive. The storefronts are distinctive and the items sold intriguing.

Yet, the levee is weak. When the river swells a bit, the levee breaks down easily. That is when the acting out occurs. I could also say that the rampart is weak, instead of the levee. Therefore, the "defense" readily collapses – not by a mighty enemy, but from even a small attack. And then the streetscape suffers damage.

Acting out and chaos

Suppose that the condition of being flooded (or invaded by the enemy) due to the levee's (or rampart's) collapse is the condition of acting out. The levee or rampart, which is weak to begin with, becomes even weaker under stress. Such clients go off and collapse even the remaining part themselves. This is the reality of the acting-out situation. People in the borderline state may feel refreshed for a moment when cutting their wrist or overdosing, but as time goes on, they begin to feel desperation: "I did it again," "how miserable," "I am totally confused," etc. People in the borderline state are already emotionally taxed, but experience even more chaotic situations by acting out. The distinctive and attractive streetscape gets ruined. The therapist, therefore, must stop their acting out in one way or another.

Not limit-setting

Preventing the acting out is not equal to limit-setting. I consider the prevention of acting out to be one of the essential psychotherapeutic factors. In a case of alcohol dependency, for instance, clients are no longer dependent on alcohol from the moment they stop drinking, regardless of the pathology. I want to introduce a perspective that considers these cases to be the same. Regardless of the pathology, acting out is itself the problem; so if acting out is stopped, people in the borderline state are presumably no longer in the borderline state. If they can restrain themselves from acting out for three years, they are close to genuine recovery. This same point applies to alcohol dependency.

Thus, my definition of the borderline case is "people not at the psychotic level (and without organic psychosis, of course) who act out." We live with various kinds of pathology. It is not unusual for this "pathology" to shape our life goals in a manner that leads us to higher possibilities. It may even give rise to great artwork. A spirit of dancing with the disease springs up. That is, the *psycheology* of dancing with madness (the shadow or wound) opens up.

I am not saying that pathology should not be questioned. What I mean is that one must reinforce the levee or rampart with sufficient strength to prevent acting out, which allows individuals to remove themselves from the borderline state in any given moment. They cannot dance without this resiliency.

People in the borderline state need to control themselves and make it through the moment – especially when they are stressed out. This is what a psychotherapist helps support. Every time they control themselves, it is like sandbags being piled up. The therapist must communicate this understanding to clients very clearly, over and over again.

A therapist must put feelings into words to stop acting out every single time

It is not an easy thing for a therapist to tell clients the same thing repeatedly and steadily. An expert, however, must at least try to do so. I saw Ichiro Suzuki[13] doing his stretching routine before a game on TV. He must have done it thousands of times. Still, he didn't cut any corners, but worked hard with steady, heartfelt effort. I think people who do quality work, regardless of their profession, are those who can do the basic routine work with this attitude. Telling clients the same thing every single time with all your heart is one of the most important "techniques."

Paternal and maternal care

To forbid acting out is an act of paternal care. There is a strictness to it. To forbid clients something they cling to for survival is a severe request. Nevertheless, this practice is simultaneously an act of maternal care that protects clients. This maternal quality in forbidding acting out must also be thoroughly understood by clients.

Offering praise

It is important for a psychotherapist to offer sufficient, heartfelt praise if clients in the borderline state are able to spend a week without acting out. I say to them, "I assume many challenging situations came up for you, yet you did a wonderful job. The levee has become that much stronger. The sandbags have piled up that much more." People in the borderline state are less likely to receive sufficient praise. They often think so, at least. Therefore, praising such clients is one of the most important techniques. Yet, it is not good to give praise about just anything. Situations impressive enough to give heartfelt praise do not occur that often. When they do, however, a therapist can praise clients from the heart, considering how they are forbidding clients from doing something that is almost impossible for them to stop.

Preventing drastic actions

I often ask my clients, "Have you done something drastic in the past week?" By something drastic I mean wrist-cutting or overdosing, although defining the range of what is considered drastic is actually difficult. It is especially difficult in the case of relationships with the opposite sex and of excessive expense on a favorite pursuit. The process of defining the range is very important, because it is also a process of shaping who they are and how that gets expressed in their lives. The difference between "what should not be done" and "the gray area" must be an ongoing discussion in therapy.

The issue of dissociation

There is, however, the issue of dissociation. Some clients say, "I cut my wrist without realizing it, so there isn't anything I can do about it." Even in such a case, I still forbid their acting out, because some part of their consciousness is working, even during dissociation. During sleep, for instance, small children fall out of bed, while adults typically do not. This is because, for adults, some part of consciousness is on duty even during sleep. Bed-wetting is the same. Even when people experience dissociative amnesia or dissociative fugue, they rarely get into traffic accidents. This is because some consciousness is on duty.

After giving this instruction to clients in the borderline state who experience dissociation, I continue, "You may not be conscious of doing these things, but it is certainly you who do it. Therefore, you are also responsible for what you do while dissociated. If you make a habit of being aware of your acting out, you will not do it even when dissociated." It is quite a strict request, as I am asking them to be responsible for themselves even during the state of dissociation, but there is more to it.

One client said, "When I wake up in the morning, there are many empty snack bags are lying around, though I have no recollection of eating. I am scared to think that I may have eaten all of them without my knowledge." Such a case is not unusual. When I shared this explanation, the client said, "I was so afraid because I thought I couldn't be helped, since I did it without knowing. I am relieved to know how to handle this." In this client's case, the problem successfully remitted.

We must also think about dissociation from another perspective.

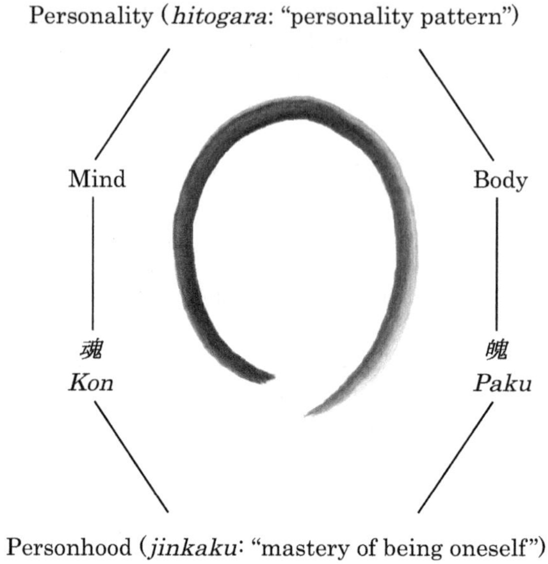

Figure 4.2

Many people don't feel any pain in wrist-cutting

The longer it takes before pain is experienced from wrist-cutting, the more difficult a case seems. At any rate, people who cut their wrists dissociate their mind from their body's pain.

There is a Japanese word, *kon-paku*[14] (魂魄; "soul"). *Kon* (魂) is believed to reside in the depths of the mind, while *paku* (魄) is believed to reside in the depths of the body. When a person dies, *kon* is believed to go to heaven, while *paku* returns to the soil. Every time people dissociate the mind from the body through wrist-cutting, *kon* and *paku* are dissociated from each other. Figure 4.2 depicts how I see this process. *Kon* and *paku* can be rejoined through the process of mastering ourselves. Others sense our whole being as our personality pattern.[15] It may look contradictory to Figure 4.1, but I consider "soul" (魂; *tamashii*) in Figure 4.1 to include *kon* (魂) and *paku* (魄) in Figure 4.2, at the center of the circle. That is how I think about it, though it may sound a bit obscure.

In addition, the dissociation in wrist-cutting has another side.

Wrist-cutting and dissociation

A client said to me, "When I see the blood after cutting my wrist, I feel relieved to realize I am alive." That is true. But realizing that one is alive by seeing red blood involves only the physical level. Mind, *kon*, and *paku* are ignored here.

In order to live for real, clients must quit acting out; otherwise, their mind and body, *kon* and *paku,* will dissociate even further. Clients cannot "dance" if they are dissociated. They will fall into chaos. Therapists must understand the suffering such clients endure, having no other choice but to act out. But they must still prevent these clients from acting out, in order to stop them from further suffering.

Therapists help clients start afresh as often as needed

There are many times when acting out does not stop right away. The explanation described above works well in some cases, but not all. What should a therapist do then? There is no choice but to start over as needed: "What is done is done. Let's start again until we get it right." That's the only choice. Stopping the acting out is not limit-setting, but rather the goal of therapy itself, so what psychotherapists and clients need to do is to keep starting over, again and again.

Once again, the streetscape

I mentioned in the previous section the fine quality of the streetscape in borderline cases; but just like any other, it is not perfect, of course.

In the case of clients in the borderline state, the garbage incinerator is not fully functioning. Many of them say, "Stress has been accumulating since childhood, and it just keeps building up. I am on the verge of dying." This is because their ability to dispose of waste is poor. Because the levee or rampart is weak, flooding or invasion by the enemy occurs and impairs certain functions. One of these functions is waste disposal.

The therapist applies the same method to this problem: constructing the levee or rampart. If clients stop acting out in extreme situations, their garbage incinerator will function better; if the town does not get flooded, construction can begin on a better treatment facility as well. At which point I say, "Let's take a lifetime to make the town more your own." This approach is valid not only for people in the borderline state, but for everyone.

Suicidal ideation

Many clients of the borderline case say they want to die. Statistics vary, but the suicide rate for borderline cases is approximately 10%. This is what therapists must remain alert to the most.

When such a client says, "I want to die," I sometimes ask, "Can you fill that out?" The ensuing dialogue often leads to the conclusion, "I want to die because I cannot do and am not doing what I want. It is a pain. I want to die." Situations of not being able to do what we want and need to do are very painful.

In fact, there are times when what clients want to do has already been done quite a lot. What is happening here is that the level of "what one wants to do" is as high as the level of seeking godhood, so people in the borderline state suffer from a sense of inability. They may be close to accomplishing it at a human level, yet those in the borderline state cannot be satisfied with this. Aiming high is not bad in itself; the problem is that the inability to make the required efforts brings suffering for such individuals, and eventually a feeling of wanting to die.

Constructing the rampart is also helpful in working with the core mental structure in the borderline state. Doing so requires efforts be made on a regular basis. Constructing the rampart means setting the "border" within them. Bringing serious harm or death to ourselves or others is a prohibited behavior for human beings. These behaviors must only be allowed by the Hand of God. Therefore, I consider prohibiting such behaviors and reinforcing the capacity to prohibit such behaviors as the real therapy.

The borderline case and its environs

Neurosis and the borderline case

The number of clients who are purely at the neurotic level has been decreasing in recent times. On the other hand, the number of people in whom neurotic and borderline processes are nearly indistinguishable has been increasing. It seems as though neuroses have taken on features resembling the borderline case. By the way, my image of neurotic people's ramparts is that they are already sufficient, but in attempting to strengthen them even more, their efforts are spoiled.

Depression and the borderline case

It has been said that the intensity of depression is becoming milder and milder, but it seems to have become closer to the borderline case as well.

Many researchers, including Masterson, have pointed out how the borderline case and depression are related. Broadly speaking, it seems to me that people are recognized as borderline if they act out, but depressed if they act in. (Acting in needs to be described more precisely, but I will not go into detail here in order to avoid complexity and confusion.) Therefore, the "border" (between depression and the borderline case) is becoming increasingly ambiguous in the mental health fields.

Schizophrenia and the borderline case

As mentioned previously, it has been questioned throughout the history of mental health whether schizophrenia and the borderline case exist on the same continuum or are independent of one another.

I'd like to share what a female client, who entered full remission of schizophrenia, said to me. "When I was really ill, I was at the center of the world. Everything, including TV and radio, was directing messages at me. I was the center, just as if I were the queen or God. Because I was queen, I was sometimes persecuted by others. People conspired to entrap me, so everyone and everything was a threat."

People in the state of personhood disorders consciously or unconsciously (in most cases half unconsciously) seek for godhood. And yet, they cannot reach the state of God. That is one reason for their suffering. However, people in the state of schizophrenia sometimes identify with God. From the perspective of godhood and personhood, there is a continuity between the state of personhood disorders and the state of schizophrenia. Nonetheless, one cannot enter the "Kingdom of God" so easily – one is rarely allowed to enter there. In that sense, there is a discontinuity as well.

What this client said was highly suggestive. Because she was in the state of queenhood, she could reject therapy. Yet, because she was in the state of queenhood, she could not escape the harsh eye of others. A therapist had better make good use of this predicament. For clients who reject taking medication because of being in the state of kinghood or queenhood, a therapist can tell them that there is a medicine that will remove their anxiety and fear. My clients often take medication if I say, "If your frustration and anxiety are that strong, you cannot fully perform your duties. It will be better first to quell your frustration and anxiety with this medicine." This proposal does not always work, especially in cases involving paranoia, which is also one of the symptoms of a king or queen. Such kings or queens sometimes arrange for a food taster.

I think that a king or queen's loneliness, anxiety, and paranoid behaviors explain the state of schizophrenia very well.

Drug and alcohol dependency and the borderline case

I consider acting out by people in the borderline state as an addiction or dependency behavior. Just as people with drug and alcohol dependency are no longer dependent once they stop taking the substances, refraining from acting out is essential in the treatment of the borderline case.

People with chronic alcoholism cannot live long. The average lifespan is little more than 50 years. One of the causes of death is suicide. Yet, it is often difficult to know whether the death is due to suicide or disease: "drinking to death,"[16] so to speak. People with alcoholism drink to forget the fact that they are drinking (just like the drinker in *The Little Prince*). In the meantime, they die amidst total chaos, both mentally and socially. This downward spiral is very similar to acting-out behaviors in the borderline case. It is only at the beginning that they feel good, whether from drinking in alcoholism or acting out in the borderline case. They soon turn to feeling badly.

It was only after the recognition of alcoholism that people began to be treated medically; before that, they were seen as not much more than "big drinkers" or "bad drinkers." What a long time it took to reach this point. It has also taken a long time to refine the treatment process for this syndrome, i.e., for clinicians to recognize that there is no choice but to quit alcohol once the alcoholic state is reached. They must quit alcohol before anything else, including psychotherapy.

Regarding acting out in the borderline case, the therapeutic theory of the borderline case could learn from the history of drug and alcohol dependency. Given the numerous clients lost to the disease, it would be downright neglectful if nothing were gleaned from the therapeutic theory of alcoholism. Some may say, "It is outrageous to discuss alcoholism and the borderline case on the same plane," but I worked at a specialized hospital for alcoholism for six years. From what I experienced there, I certainly believe that my recognition of the acting out by the borderline case as an addictive behavior is not wrong.

Treatment of the borderline case

The fragmentation of the public spirit (*seken*)[17] is a modern phenomenon in Japan. For better or worse, these tacit social rules apart from the law are shattered nowadays. As a result, it is getting more and more difficult for people to contain their thoughts and behaviors. The mental mechanisms of seeking for godhood are becoming activated with increasing ease. This tendency is similar to problems that were brought on by the fragmentation of God in Christianity. Holding this context in mind, let's take a closer look at what arises in therapy.

The state of personhood trait dysfunction

As mentioned before, the assumption that prohibiting clients from acting out stresses them and may trigger suicide is incorrect in a lot of cases. Rather, it eases them (the prohibition must clearly communicate maternal care, of course). Preventing clients from acting out is definitely the right thing to do, but one must be well aware of how the "right thing" can also be destructive. When it seems to be a type of borderline case that is an extension of hysteria, doing this is entirely possible. When a case seems to be trending towards schizophrenia, however, a therapist must work very carefully.

I am not certain enough to generalize, but I think a therapist must be alert if people in the borderline state are very affable. Such clients appear to be agreeable when they should be mentally weighed down. This agreeableness is a bit different than trying to be a good person. It seems to represent a dysfunction. The character traits of such individuals are expressed too little. Generally, when people's traits come through, their unique pattern[18] can be sensed by others; but in cases of agreeable borderline people, the expression of their traits is diminished. Thus, such individuals experience a state of "personhood trait dysfunction"[19] that affects their capacity to be unique individuals or characters, and they require additional support.

There is a drawing pattern for the tree in the Baum Test that agreeable borderline people compose that I call the "amoeba trunk." The form of the tree trunk is so indefinite that it gives an impression not unlike an amoeba. When the state is less dysfunctional, the form of the trunk is vertically symmetrical; it is still a bit amoeba-like, but the trunk looks almost identical if flipped upside down.

Being appreciated

There are some cases in which I get criticized or attacked by clients. That is not easy, but I can understand it when I perceive their situations.

However, what if I am appreciated by clients? It is fine when the appreciation fits the situation, but if not, therapists must be alert. In the worst case, clients may have come to say goodbye. Or if the present condition is too difficult, it may be that they cannot help projecting an overly idealized image onto the therapist, saying, "What a wonderful therapist!" If the therapist considers it necessary to devalue this and says, "No, I am just doing this as a paid job," clients may be endangered because such words may suddenly wash away their mirage, thus removing a fragile support. It is sometimes necessary for therapists to accept and play the part of a wonderful therapist.

It is also necessary for therapists to be sensitive when receiving gifts. It is probably okay to accept most presents, but the problem is how to handle them once they have been received. It depends on various things, but throwing away or treating poorly what is supposed to be treasured may increase the likelihood of trouble.[20] A therapist, therefore, must think through this issue carefully.

A state of affinity for "evil"

Though not limited to them, I have the impression that people in the borderline state (and particularly those in the severe range) appear to encounter extraordinary situations more frequently. They encounter one thing after another – like encountering the scene of someone's suicide or witnessing a traffic accident – in a manner befitting the phrase "accident-prone." They seem to encounter reflections of their internal mental conflicts or heartrending sorrows in externalized forms in the physical world. That is my impression.

When I see such clients, I listen to what happened to them in the same mode as when I listen to dreams. That way, I can see their suffering a bit more clearly. People who often encounter extraordinary events are somehow on the same wavelength as these extraordinary matters, and their inner state is equally terrible in its turmoil. Such cases are also addressed by supporting the construction of the rampart. Distancing oneself from such extraordinary events requires considerable energy. Thus, therapists support clients' attempts to build up their own energy. If therapists and clients work together, clients' wavelengths begin to shift out of the register of extraordinary matters little by little.

Deeds

Therapists must help clients become who they are. It is always clients who play the major role in therapy.

People accomplish deeds in order to become themselves. I don't say a behavior because a deed includes more than external actions. For instance, restraining an urge to cut one's wrist is a deed. Without deeds, it is impossible to construct the levee, the rampart, or the town. Therefore, therapists must be sensitive to the deeds clients are attempting and accomplishing. As a means to this end, I sometimes ask clients about their dreams, and other times ask them to draw pictures.

Psychopathy here again

As mentioned before, the study of personhood disorders was preceded by the study of psychopathy. Let's take another look at psychopathy.

Schneider lamented the extinction of the psychopathy concept. So do I. In an interesting twist, the term psychopath has instead become a household word. Cruel and brutal people, like Hannibal Lecter in the movie *The Silence of the Lambs*, are called psychopaths. While the term has disappeared from mental health, the concept continues to carry quite a lively image.

Now, everything has both positive and negative sides, but can there really be any positive side to psychopathy?

Tragedies abound in this world. In most cases, there is no real explanation. It's as though they are brutal attacks by the psychopathy of the world. Some things, however, cannot be activated without such attacks.

Jesus Christ said to "pray for those who persecute you" (Matthew 5:44, New International Version), but what did He mean? Let's think about it by putting "those who persecute you" into "extraordinary situations" that would provide the tremendous energy required for an individuation process that would not become activated but for these extraordinary situations (C. G. Jung). If we could at all view such situations in this way – and survive them – the unchangeable past would begin to change. If we could face forward with a prayer even when caught in stone-cold and unexplainably psychopathic situations, the past could change for us, although the factual past would not change. It may not be until then that psychopathy dies and we can be born again.

Notes

1 Translators' note: In this work, *jinkaku-shōgai* is translated as "personhood disorder" and *personality-shōgai* is translated as "personality disorder." The author's preference for the former term is described below.
2 Translators' note: *Jinkaku*: personality; *shōgai*: "disorder." The literal meaning of the Chinese characters composing *jinkaku* (人格) signify the rank, style, or rule of a person.
3 Translators' note: *Hito*: person; *gara*: decorative pattern.
4 Translators' note: As is discussed in the Conclusion, the Japanese are subject to the strictures of both society and the public spirit (*seken*). The responsibilities associated with maintaining these strictures rest primarily with the mature adult population (i.e., those above age 40). What the author is implying here is that when the traditional therapeutic method is used (i.e., the focus is not on reducing clients' acting out), treatment takes much longer. Thus, a situation can arise in which adolescents with borderline personality disorder may be in treatment sufficiently long that, as adults, they no longer meet diagnostic criteria – not so much because treatment was effective, but because the strictures of society and the public spirit constrain their acting out as mature adults more than when they were younger.
5 Translators' note: *Jin*: person.
6 Translators' note: 神格 (神, *shin*: God; 格, *kaku*: to master). 神 means "God" and has two pronunciations: *shin, kami*. Since Chinese characters were imported to Japan, there are two manners of referring to them in Japanese: *on-yomi* and

kun-yomi. *On-yomi* represents the Chinese pronunciation, while *kun-yomi* represents the pre-existing Japanese oral language. The *on-yomi* of 神 is *shin* or *jin*, and the *kun-yomi* is *kami*, *kan*, or *kou*.

7 Translators' note: Morel's theory argued that Adam's original sin began the inevitable degeneration of the human race. While this degeneration bore upon all of humanity, eventually leading to sterility and extinction, Morel nevertheless believed the rate of decline was open to influence. As a result, some individuals might suffer greater degenerative effects than others.

8 Translators' note: A superior degenerate is one in whom all of the mental faculties may be developed to a degree greater than average, yet are unbalanced amongst themselves in a manner that gives rise to emotional imbalance, mental discord, and even derangement (Hirsch, 1897, pp. 125–126).

9 Translators' note: A useful summary of each type is provided in Millon's *Disorders of Personality* (2011). The descriptions for the hyperthymic, affectionless, and asthenic types follow:

"Hyperthymic personalities reflect a mix of high activity, optimism, and shallowness; they tend to be uncritical, cocksure, impulsive, and undependable. Many seem unable to concentrate, and those who achieve occasional insights fail to retain them as lasting impressions" (p. 12).

"Affectionless personalities lack compassion and are often considered callous and cold; they appear distant or indifferent to friends and strangers alike. Historically, these patients correspond to those identified in the literature as exhibiting 'moral insanity'" (p. 12).

"[T]he asthenic personality, subjects him- or herself to intense hypochondriacal scrutiny and is so preoccupied with bodily functions that external events fade into the background and appear strange or unreal" (pp. 12–13).

10 Translators' note: The date of the work is simply noted here and is not intended to indicate a citation.

11 Translators' note: As discussed at further length in the Translators' introduction, the original publication of this work predates DSM-5. This translation thus reflects the DSM-IV-TR model and nomenclature except where otherwise specified.

12 Translators' note: In the Japanese juvenile corrections system, a classification home is focused on assessing juveniles in order to make appropriate recommendations for subsequent services.

13 Translators' note: A Japanese baseball player.

14 Translators' note: In Japanese, the kanji character 魂 can be spoken as either *kon* or *tamashii* but has the identical meaning of "soul." *Kon-paku* refers to a Chinese concept that was imported into Japanese, the significance of which is described by the author in this paragraph. *Kon-paku* might be thought of as an elaboration on the term *tamashii* discussed earlier in the chapter.

15 Translators' note: *Hitogara*. *Hito*: person; *gara*: pattern. It refers to a very subtle, intuitive sense of a person. There is a certain commonality with the tendency in English to use flavor words to describe someone's personality: sweet, tart, bitter, etc. *Hitogara* represents a similar but subtler version of this.

16 Translators' note: In Japanese, this phrase represents a new coinage by the author.

17 Translators' note: *Seken* is a term distinctive to Japanese culture. Roughly translated, *seken* means "world around you." It has also been translated as "world," "society," "public," or "life." Here, it is translated as "public spirit."

Seken originated as a Buddhist term for all the living things and elements surrounding us. In terms of daily experience, *seken* signifies a given individual's sphere of interpersonal concern. It varies from person to person, but generally involves several concentric rings of social influence: from family, to the people with whom one often has contact, to the broader social sphere.

18 Translators' note: Or, as discussed in a previous endnote, their "flavor." In other words, one can get a "feel" for the person as a whole, or what they are like.

19 Translators' note: In Japanese, this phrase represents a new coinage by the author.

20 Translators' note: In the Japanese Shinto tradition, *kami* or gods are believed to reside in various objects. The implication is that a *kami* residing in the gifted object might retaliate.

21 Translators' note: A number of the sources noted here were not directly cited in the text, but rather served as general sources for the information presented: (Kato, Kasahara, Okonogi, Hozaki, & Miyamoto, 1993; Ohigashi, 1999; Sadock & Sadoci, 2000; Seishin-igaku Kōza Tantousha-kaigi, 1998; Ujihara, Narita, Higashiyama, Kameguchi, & Yamanaka, 2004).

References

Akita, I. (2000). Henro-to-sonzai-in [Pilgrimage and the cause of existence]. *Psyche, 19*, 120–127.

Akita, I. (2011). Shinkeisho-to-seishinbyo [Neurosis and psychosis] (II). In The Association of Japanese Clinical Psychology (Ed.), *Shinri-rinshōgaku-jiten* [Encyclopedia of clinical psychology] (pp. 244–245). Tokyo, Japan: Maruzen-Shuppan.

American Psychiatric Association (1980). *Diagnostic and statistical manual of mental disorders* (3rd ed.). Washington, DC: Author.

American Psychiatric Association (1995). *Diagnostic and statistical manual of mental disorders* (4th ed., S. Takahashi, Y. Oono, & T. Someya, Trans.). Tokyo, Japan: Igaku Shoin.

American Psychiatric Association (2000). *Diagnostic and statistical manual of mental disorders* (4th ed., text revision). Washington, DC: Author.

American Psychiatric Association (2002). *Diagnostic and statistical manual of mental disorders* (4th ed., text revision, S. Takahashi, Y. Oono, & T. Someya, Trans.). Tokyo, Japan: Igaku Shoin.

Hayashi, N. (2005). *Personality-shōgai* [Personality disorders]. Tokyo, Japan: Shinko Igaku Shuppan.

Hirsch, W. (1897). *Genius and degeneration: A psychological study.* Retrieved from https://archive.org/details/geniusdegenerati00hirs

Kato, M., Kasahara, Y., Okonogi, K., Hozaki, H., & Miyamoto, T. (Eds.) (1993). *Shinpan seishin igaku jiten* [Encyclopedia of psychiatric medicine, new edition]. Tokyo, Japan: Koubundo.[21]

Millon, T. (2011). *Disorders of personality: Introducing a DSM/ICD spectrum from normal to abnormal* (3rd ed.). Hoboken, NJ: Wiley.

Nishiyama, A. (2004). Seishin-byoushitsuron-no-yukue [Trace of psychopathy]. In K. Takaoka & T. Okamura (Eds.), *Mental health library: Vol. 11. Emergence labelled personality disorders: Theoretical disputes* (pp. 134–150). Tokyo, Japan: Hihansha.

Ohigashi, Y. (1999). Morel-to-Magnan: Henshitsuron-no-yukue [Morel and Magnan: The track of the theory of degeneration]. In A. Fujinawa, Y. Ohigashi, & K.

Shingu (Eds.), *Seishinigaku-gunzo* [Psychiatric medicine group] (pp. 125–144). Kyoto, Japan: Academia Shuppankai.

Okada, T. (2005). *Kodaijiko-shoukougun* [Grandiose self syndrome]. Tokyo, Japan: Chikuma Shobo.

Ootsuki, S. (1978). *Seishin-igaku* [Psychiatric medicine] (pp. 248–253). Tokyo, Japan: Bunkoudo.

Sadock, B. J. & Sadoci, V. A. (Eds.) (2000). *Kaplan & Sadock's comprehensive textbook of psychiatry* (7th ed., Vols. 1–2). Philadelphia, PA: Lippincott Williams & Wilkins.

Seishin-igaku Kōza Tantousha-kaigi [Psychiatric Medicine Course Committee] (Ed.) (1998). *Senmoni-wo-mezasuhitono-seishin-igaku* [Psychiatric medicine for those who aspire to become specialized physicians]. Tokyo, Japan: Igaku Shoin.

Ujihara, H., Narita, Y., Higashiyama, H., Kameguchi, K., & Yamanaka, Y. (Eds.) (2004). *Shinri-rinshō-daijiten* [Encyclopedia of psychotherapy]. Tokyo, Japan: Baifukan.

World Health Organization (1993). *The ICD-10 classification of mental and behavioural disorders: Clinical descriptions and diagnostic guidelines* (M. Tooru, Y. Nakane, & M. Komiyama, Trans.). Tokyo, Japan: Igaku Shoin.

Chapter 5

For those who wander in mazes

Escaping the fly bottle

At the end of Chapter 4, I mentioned the psychopathy of the world. There are many phenomena that are indescribable without the use of such language. When the world, God, heaven, or the universe suddenly shows its fangs, we paltry humans cannot explain such situations, but resort to describing them as attacks by the psychopathy of the world.

The question of "why" arises in such situations. On March 11, 2011, for instance, why did people living in the Tōhoku and Kantō regions have to fall victim to the massive earthquake? As mentioned, it can be easily explained as a "how" question; it was only the plate movement that occurred off the coast of the Tōhoku region.

The answer to the question, "Why is this happening to me?," however, cannot be answered. The only way left is to dance the suffering with the *cause of existence*. In other words, "I" and "psychopathy," which have existed separately, must begin to dance together, just like the double-helical structure of DNA. Or one must live out the *disfigured hero* archetype. While it may not seem at all seismic when viewed from without, but rather a minor event, it can be a major tremor for the person in question. Some may choose death, it is so difficult to continue living.

To add some points regarding "why" questions, a person's attitude in confronting them generally becomes quieter and deeper with maturity. However, people in the borderline state act out the questions themselves.[1] In contrast, people with schizophrenia are sometimes completely locked up in such questions.[2]

"Why" questions are easily brought up for people in the borderline state over the littlest things, like a partner emailing five minutes later than the promised time. "Why? Despite my waiting for so long. . . ." The range of "why" questions is quite broad for people in the borderline state. (Constructing the rampart or the levee is also effective here. They will eventually be able to hold on amidst the rampant "why" questions.)

For people with schizophrenia, the rampant "why" questions become a maze that locks them up. The issue of mazes is not limited to schizophrenia:

mazes sometimes appear in the dreams of people with serious depression. One of my clients frequently dreams about a maze. He is locked up in the maze and cannot get out. In addition, the maze itself moves – a transforming maze. A regular maze is already complicated to get out of, but despair creeps in if the maze itself transforms.

Individuals can remain at the level of personhood disorders as long as the "why" questions run rampant in or with them. If, however, their running rampant begins to lock up the self, they will shift into a state of psychosis.

I began to have an interest in mazes when I was writing "A Study on the Disfigured Hero" (2001). I compared various aspects of the West with Japan, and in doing so, was by struck by the realization that mazes in the West and Japan are very different. While the Western maze has its goal in the middle, the Japanese maze has its exit (goal) independent of its entrance: one wanders in at one point and exits somewhere else. Ever since I noticed the difference, I have been pointing out issues from the perspective of mazes in my lectures and seminars at Kyoto Bunkyo University and in the group supervision at the Association of Jungian Analysts, Japan. Also, in the undergraduate course on dream analysis at Kyoto Bunkyo University, I set "maze or repetition" as the initial topic. (Repetition is considered to be a type of a maze.)

Symbolization

I would like to briefly introduce the theory of the *disfigured hero*.

In the West, there exist few wounded heroes like Black Jack.[3] When wounded, a character in the West typically becomes a monster who then plays a sacrificial role for the individuation of the hero character. In contrast, a character in Japan can attain the *disfigured hero* image, so to speak: Zatōichi, Tange Sazen, Captain Harlock, Queen Emeraldas,[4] Kenshiro from the *manga First of the North Star*, Guts from *Berserk*, etc. Such individuals begin to shine out even more once "disfigured." A special talent, which can only be performed by the disfigured prodigy, emerges.

Why can disfigured characters shine out in Japan? One answer is that the idea of two heroes standing abreast is deeply ingrained in Japanese culture. That is, ego and shadow (or the prior life and the scar) stand abreast. This dynamism is firmly rooted in the culture. They are not reduced to monsters even if disfigured, but rather, can become heroes. They do not have to be heroes, but if they continue to live fully even after being deeply wounded, the ego and the shadow become intertwined like the double-helical structure of DNA and elaborate who they are. In some cases, they become heroic as a result.

In the West, the shadow is considered that which must be integrated into the ego; in other words, the devil must be disempowered before God. Is seeing the shadow from such a perspective also adequate for Japan? I won't go into detail, but I want to introduce the idea of *psycheology* dancing with shadow here. My point is that in the course of the ego intertwining with the shadow, which is reflected in a wound or madness, such individuals begin to exert the unique attractiveness and talent that only they can express.

The manner in which the shadow, a wound, or madness can give rise to "dancing madness" has been depicted with sublime beauty in the classical Japanese performing arts, especially *Noh, Kabuki, and Bunraku.* I will touch upon this point a little at the end of this book, and hope to discuss it further at another time.

Black Jack is the figure I place at the top of the pack for *disfigured heroes.*

This is because, in Japan, there are a number of heroes whose images become more attractive due to a wound, but most of them use their power and attractiveness to fight, i.e., to eliminate their opponents. Black Jack, however, uses the power and attraction he gained from being wounded, and living through that hardship, to save the lives of others. By remaining grounded, he never lets himself use his ability for revenge, though the temptation can be strong. To explain the storyline, Black Jack and his mother were seriously injured by five criminals. Black Jack did retaliate against the first criminal (Episode 115, 1976/1987). With the second criminal, however, Black Jack held himself back as best he could (Episode 195, 1977/1988). This was when Black Jack, who did not use his power for revenge, reached completion.

One student said to me, "There have been many heroes who didn't seek revenge but tried to heal people, though deeply wounded, such as Hōnen.[5] Black Jack is not the only wounded hero." I replied that there have surely been many outstanding individuals, but becoming a symbolic image is another matter.

There are many people who are as brave as Don Quixote, standing up against the strong without regard for their own raw power. What was remarkable about Cervantes, however, was his brilliant symbolization of such individuals though the figure of Don Quixote, who challenged windmills to duels. Perhaps there are also many who have been as intensely self-sacrificing as Jesus Christ. But it was Jesus who became symbolized through the image of Christ on the cross. Christianity gained enough influence to spread all over the world, in both positive and negative ways, by achieving this symbolization. It lies at the root of Christianity.

It is the same with Black Jack. There may exist many prominent people who do not use their special abilities for revenge, despite having been wounded and gaining power. Osamu Tezuka, the author of *Black Jack*, successfully symbolized these people through Black Jack. It is not a question of who is superior, Hōnen or Black Jack. Rather, it is in this symbolization that the greatness of Osamu Tezuka can be found.

The image and symbol of a maze

This is also the way of things with mazes. We are all in doubt and distressed. We all bumble and stumble through life, probably without exception. When doubt and distress become serious, people feel as though they have lost their sense of direction, their egos have collapsed, or they have been locked up. All of these sensations are similar to being locked up in a maze. Some genius of times past symbolized this powerful influence on the human experience through mazes.

There do exist a variety of real mazes, such as simple mazes for children; the turf mazes and hedge mazes seen mainly in the U.K. (the oldest existing hedge maze was built in 1690 and is preserved in the garden of Hampton Court Palace); the stone labyrinths in Scandinavian countries; the pavement labyrinths in the Gothic cathedrals, such as at Chartres and Notre Dame; etc. These are materialized mazes or labyrinths, but the source of such real mazes or labyrinths is the sensation of inescapable suffering that exists in our minds. The sense of being locked up in a prison has become an image of a maze or labyrinth, and it has come to appear frequently in mythology, legend, and also reality.

Mazes in the West

> The pattern of labyrinths from ancient times to the medieval era is characterized by a singular pathway structure, without any splits or choices, that winds around thoroughly inside of the figure . . . But after the Baroque period (17th century), the pattern of labyrinths gradually lost their original mystic quality, while their playful characteristics were strengthened with the intention to trick.
>
> (Yokoyama, 1988, p. 13, our translation)

Labyrinths are generally recognized to have one pathway, while mazes have splits. There is no difference, however, with respect to their essence of locking in. You may wonder how one gets lost on a singular pathway. Here is what happens.

If you go into a labyrinth without a map, you do not know whether the pathway is singular or not, just like the labyrinth Daedalus built in Knossos. Described as a pathway that "winds around thoroughly," the labyrinth disorients you in the course of walking around. Eventually you lose your sense of direction entirely and get caught up in fear and despair. Therefore, it is extremely difficult for a person in a labyrinth to recognize that there is only one pathway.

The labyrinth of Knossos Palace is called the Cretan labyrinth pattern, as it is located in Crete. The Minotaur, a monster with the head of a bull on the body of a man, was born to a bull and Pasiphaë, the wife of the Cretan King Minos, and was locked up in the labyrinth that Daedalus built inside Knossos Palace. The chronological order of events in this famous story was that first the monster existed, and then it was locked up. The essence, however, is that one becomes monstrous if kept locked up in a maze or labyrinth – or both could happen simultaneously. This is another fundamental pathology involved with the state of serious personhood disorders or psychosis.

Mazes in the West are center-oriented. In other words, the state of being locked up in the deepest spot is "pursued." If people remain in the state of being locked up in the depths, they become monstrous beyond the point of recognition.

> Within a medieval Christian context, the Chartres labyrinth possesses an especially rich symbolism. To begin with, its 11 concentric circular paths (the Cretan labyrinth had seven) reflect a well-developed number symbolism. The number 11 stands for sin, for it oversteps boundaries (10 marks a boundary within the decimal system). Moreover, it is an imperfect number, being one more than the Ten Commandments and one less than the 12 apostles. The 11 circles of the labyrinth may have been taken to represent the *orbus peccatus*, or "world of sin."
>
> (Moon, 1997, p. 67)

Chartres Labyrinth appears to be divided into a quadrant if viewed from above, with the two orthogonal lines forming a cross. "Placed over the 'world of sin,' the cross performs a redemptive function" (p. 67). By overlapping the cross onto the ancient labyrinth, "the meaning of the entire pattern is transformed: no longer is the Devil or the Minotaur at its center, but heaven or Jerusalem."

Ancient mazes and labyrinths were oriented to a monster. Christian mazes and labyrinths were also oriented to the center, but the center meant the Virgin Mary, Christ, and the holy city of Jerusalem. In other words, Chartres Labyrinth is oriented to God. Therefore, the joy of reaching the center must be overwhelming. A maze is related to "amaze," the sense of being overwhelmed with wonder. Such joy must include intense feelings of astonishment, ecstasy, or numen. Combining the light with the joy, however, is probably too bright. One should not stay there for long: basking too long in the glory of reaching the center can make one monstrous. Godhood, the other side of being monstrous, penetrates one too much. One's personhood then falls into a state of dysfunction.

Encountering a monster is frightening, while encountering God is numinous. But they are essentially one. "Negative numen" is emphasized in the Cretan Labyrinth, while "positive numen" is emphasized in the Chartres Labyrinth. Even though the feeling is positive, we should not stay there for long. Because both numena are one, both will ultimately penetrate our being with too much intensity. It is better to hold onto the joy as a momentary one to be treasured for the rest of our lives. The ecstasy must be momentary.

For the Japanese, who are good at carving out moments, keeping the ecstatic joy as momentary is not extremely difficult – though not easy, either. This Japanese way of carving out moments and expressing them in poetry called *haiku* or *tanka* can be useful here. The reason why the Japanese like to take photographs might also be related.

How about in the clinical practice of psychiatry? Five-minute consultations are typical in Japan. Fifteen or 20 minutes at least are necessary for consultations, but these five-minute consultations can manage the situation in some wise, perhaps because the Japanese are able to work collaboratively, in complete accord, and are good at holding "moments" in their minds. It may be because some kind of "*haiku* without words" is shared between a psychiatrist and a client, although no *haiku* or *tanka* is actually written in clinical practice. Western clients sometimes visit me, but this accord does not happen. Of course, my inadequate language skills play a role, but I assume the five-minute consultation would be impossible even if I could speak English like a native. Such a sense of *haiku* does not work with these Western clients. The situation may change, however, as *haiku* has become increasingly popular in the West; but it is going to be a long time before that change occurs.

Speaking of collaborative work, when the major earthquake mentioned above hit Japan in 2011, there were no large-scale riots or robberies (although minor riots and robberies might have occurred). Friends of mine from abroad, including Australia, the United Kingdom, Switzerland, the United States, and Taiwan, shared praise such as, "It is only the Japanese who can collaborate and help each other in complete accord even in the midst of such a disaster." I was studying in Switzerland when the Great Hanshin-Awaji Earthquake[6] occurred, but my mentor, Guggenbühl-Craig, said, "The *Yakuza* were passing buckets filled with water to extinguish the fire. The mafia in the West would never do such things."

However, when I dropped my contact lens at the airport in Switzerland, about six people realized the situation, and, to my surprise, gathered around me and tried to search for it. Such a scene is unfortunately quite rare in Japan.

The Japanese support each other in major disasters, but cannot in minor ones. Can the Japanese spirit of harmony not be activated except in extreme circumstances? Mental health practice is full of major disasters. Clients sit tentatively in the waiting room like lambs, though their minds are as chaotic as major disasters. That may be why the collaborative work can take place. A clinician should not forget the fact that clients are in the midst of major disasters.

It should also not be overlooked that all *disfigured heroes* are those who have suffered from major disasters. This archetype is not activated by minor disasters.

Let's return to the topic of mazes and labyrinths.

Escape

Does a person remain locked up for good, or is it possible to get out of a maze?

Escape can be easy and difficult at the same time. In other words, changing one's awareness a little bit would make for an easy escape, but that little bit of change is quite burdensome.

To return to the Cretan Labyrinth in Knossos Palace, it was King Minos who locked up Daedalus (who built this labyrinth) and his son, Icarus, in the labyrinth. What King Minos could not forgive was Daedalus making a statue of the bull for Pasiphaë. Despite being the inventor of the labyrinth himself, Daedalus could not escape from it. As mentioned before, whether a pathway is singular or has splits, the essence of mazes and labyrinths is the impossibility of escape.

In labyrinths, one cannot successfully complete the path despite its being singular. If seen from above, the person swings back and forth inside the labyrinth like a pendulum, unable to make progress. It symbolizes with precision the suffering of being locked up, such as in the state of personhood disorders.

In the case of mazes, where the pathway has splits, one must decide which way to go. It is interesting to note that a number of people in the state of personhood disorders are not good at choosing. They have a particularly difficult time choosing between two options. They can narrow a number of possibilities down to two choices, but they cannot pick one over the other. Even when they can choose, they experience it as the only crummy possibility available to them. They don't know the importance of giving up the other choice. They cannot stand this situation. They don't yet understand that the chosen pathway, which has opened up only after letting go of the other option, will begin to shine. "Wandering" is one of the deep pathologies of people in the state of personhood disorders.

Given that the essence of mazes and labyrinths is the impossibility of escape, labyrinths that served as pilgrimages in medieval Europe do not constitute labyrinths in our sense of the term. If one drops the knee and follows the route, one can reach the goal by divine guidance, as well as return to the original point. This is because one knows from the beginning that the pathway is singular, and thus escapable. One knows that the pathway is just a complicated singular way.

Similarly, *Shikoku Henro*[7] (pilgrimage) in Japan does not have a maze-like characteristic, though it is a religious ritual or discipline. There is the divine guidance in the labyrinths of Christian churches, while the (Japanese) pilgrim's staff is considered to be Kūkai[8] in pilgrimages. Given this perspective, labyrinths in Christian churches would be more appropriately termed miniature pilgrimages by their nature: a labyrinth in shape, a miniature pilgrimage in essence.

Henro (pilgrimage) can also be considered as one of the Japanese psychotherapies. I have been pointing out therapists' slight presence as a characteristic of Japanese psychotherapies for some decades, and *henro* (pilgrimage) is one example in point. The pilgrims' attitude of walking along with the pilgrims' staff – though with Kūkai, who accompanies them – emphasizes the attitude of walking on their own. In Morita Therapy and Naikan Therapy,[9] both of which originated in Japan, therapists' involvement is less active than in Western counseling. There are probably reasons for this. As I wrote in another article, "The Japanese, who lack a sense of collective 'sin' or reject it, have no choice but to face an extremely personal process of individuation" (1997, p. 25, our translation). Yet, people also walk around the labyrinths incorporated into the floors of Western Christian churches on their own with the help of Providence. You can see the "slight presence" of therapists here. This example allows us to infer that an attitude similar to that of the Japanese psychotherapies existed in the West prior to the advent of modern Western psychotherapy.

Let's return once again to the labyrinth in Knossos Palace. Daedalus and Icarus were able to escape from it, not by walking along the winding path, but with Daedalus' brilliantly crafted wings. They became like birds, escaping the labyrinth through flight, though young Icarus flew too high and was killed in the fall.

What Daedalus did was to create a three-dimensional world by adding one more dimension to the two-dimensional one. He changed the dimension.

Changing the dimension is a necessary task for people who do not have Ariadne's clew. Mazes and labyrinths can serve a symbolic function, even if they don't exist in the real world. All mazes or labyrinths are generated in the depths of our own minds, following the pattern of the maze archetype, so to speak. If we see the current situation as a maze, it becomes a maze. The stronger we believe it to be so, the more maze-like the situation becomes. This is the situation where we get locked up. This situation can be described as the state of personhood disorders, and if it becomes more serious, we will reach the state of psychosis.

People in the state of personhood disorders suffer from being locked up. They run about in confusion. On the other hand, people in the state of psychosis are more strongly locked up, but they don't run about – they can't. If they ran about, their inner maze, which is strongly internalized, would itself act up.

Mazes or labyrinths are created by our subjective viewpoint. Thus, once another subjective viewpoint – a new perspective – is acquired, the maze or labyrinth disappears in an instant. Our subjective viewpoints are sufficiently powerful to make this happen. Magical items like Aladdin's lamp are probably images of the great power our subjective viewpoints have.

I always say that one of the purposes of clinical psychology is to provide us with wider and deeper perspectives of the world, which in turn provide us with an enhanced ability to change the dimension. Commonsensically, this can also be phrased as helping clients gain multiple perspectives that allow them to see things from various directions.

Ryōma Sakamoto[10] said, "There is not one, but hundreds and thousands of ways to live" (Shiba, 1962–1966/1998, p. 197, our translation). These words capture Sakamoto's genius for changing the dimension. We would no longer be locked up in a maze if we reached this level. Paradoxically, once we recognize that there are "hundreds and thousands of ways," the situation is no longer a maze. "One way" becomes rather mazy and locks us up. That is what is frightening about the labyrinth's singular way.

In a worldview that aspires towards Almighty God, the risk of getting locked up deep in the midst of things is high. The mazes of the West are strong bastilles, and serve that function. On the other hand, the mazes of Japan have less power to keep us locked up. The function is less mazy and more open because of the structure; that is, we enter from somewhere and exit somewhere else. In Japan, there is no story like that of the Minotaur locked up in the Labyrinth of Knossos to symbolize a fear of mazes and labyrinths. A symbolic implication of this is that the Japanese may be relatively less subject to getting locked up.

Western people have strong egos. Although I cannot immediately conclude that their egos are at the center of their labyrinths, I have observed a difference in how Westerners and the Japanese depict the mind in pictorial form: depth psychologists from the West tend to draw a closed circle, while a circle whose bottom is open is often used in Japan. The framework becomes clearer and stronger by being locked up. Therefore, we should not forget the possibility that the stronger one's mind, the more locked up in a situation one is without recognizing it.

If this is the case, what makes it possible for the Japanese to be locked up less frequently? A capacity and power to live with the wound. As mentioned, however, this wound must be somewhat deep. Shallow wounds are unlikely to activate the individuation process for the Japanese because there is no "foundation" to serve as a starting point. The wound must be deep enough to reach the core of one's existence.

And what has given rise to Westerners being locked up more strongly? One response can be found in Christ after the crucifixion.

Christ after the crucifixion

The worst misfortune to befall the West is probably the fact that Jesus Christ did not remain in this world. In other words, the greatest shortcoming of the Bible is that it does not fully depict Jesus Christ after the crucifixion. Born in Bethlehem and called Jesus of Nazareth, Jesus Christ preached, suffered on the cross, died, and was resurrected. But He did not stay here. He ascended into Heaven.

Christ was suffering on the cross: whipped, wounded by the crown of thorns, His hands and feet pierced by nails, bleeding, and His side pierced with a spear. The excruciating pain He endured to redeem everyone's sins is presented in cruel, gruesome detail. As a result, the image of Christ suffering on the cross accomplishes an incomparably high level of symbolization. Containing almost all emotions, from despair to delight, He stood with dignity despite the pain.

This was the peak of "Jesus Christ." He reached this extreme and brought the symbol to completion.

Because of this completion, Christ after the crucifixion – Christ living the wound – could not exist, and this has proven to be a negative legacy for posterity. People whose sins were forgiven through the Passion were simultaneously burdened with a significant task. Nay, they lost the task – the burden – to burden. "*Eli, Eli, lema sabachthani?* (My God, my God, why have you forsaken me?)" (Matthew 27:46, New International Version).

He was forsaken by God and wounded – and then what?

"Come to me, all you who are weary and burdened, and I will give you rest" (Matthew 11:28). This is Christ's well-known phrase, but please read it again slowly. It is just a collection of printed words, yet it really gives us rest. It has a power that can soak into the folds of deep suffering. It is miraculous. That is God's Word. However, they are the words of Jesus before the crucifixion.

It is after being burdened with their own "crosses" that people suffer greatly. That is why I want to hear His words, not written in the Bible, after His crucifixion.

Two thousand years later, *Black Jack* appeared. The work of Christ was passed on "where the ring of time is linked afar"[11] (Matsumoto, 1990, p. 340, our translation). Osamu Tezuka, a rare genius, made this possible.

Black Jack was beaten miserably and burdened with unreasonable wounds. He nevertheless came to accept this injustice with his whole being, at which point these wounds shone out and marked his existence. There may be no other figure that represents the possibility of this transition as masterfully as Black Jack. The course of how the Black Jack image was formed is a miracle.

Escaping the fly bottle

It was in my undergraduate days when I first learned of the philosopher Wittgenstein. A friend introduced me to a book written by Tetsurou Morimoto,[12] and I have since read almost all of his books. In Morimoto's book, *Journey to Words* (1978), Wittgenstein was introduced in the chapter entitled "About Philosophy."

Morimoto wrote, "Thus, philosophers were at loss in the labyrinth of words," and then quoted the words of Wittgenstein: "What is your aim in philosophy? To show the fly the way out of the fly-bottle" (p. 60, our translation).

This allegorical phrase has a subtle impact that is simple yet frightening. The tone of this philosophy is somewhat similar to my friend himself. I have often quoted this phrase since becoming a student of clinical psychology,[13] and stated that my purpose in clinical psychology was the very same.

I wouldn't dare say that I completely understand Wittgenstein's philosophy. Wittgenstein thought that even Bertrand Russell, who was his teacher, couldn't understand him. Russell wrote an introduction to Wittgenstein's book, *Tractatus Logico-Philosophicus*, but Wittgenstein was so upset that he didn't want the book published if such an introduction were to accompany it. I can never fully understand such a philosophy that was incomprehensible even for the teacher.

This quote from Wittgenstein is powerful nevertheless. It is like the way in which you can instantly grasp the archetypal aspect of Don Quixote simply by knowing the image of a man who challenged windmills, without reading the whole book. The quote carries such a rich symbolism. Relying on its symbolic power, I say once again that the purpose with my *psycheology* is to help people find their way out of mazes and labyrinths.

Notes

1 Translators' note: i.e., in response to the rampant "why" questions presenting themselves, such individuals react quickly, without reflection, and thus act them out (externalize).

2 Translators' note: i.e., in response to the rampant "why" questions presenting themselves, such individuals are overwhelmed and shut down (internalize).

3 Translators' note: Main character from a Japanese *manga*, *Black Jack*. Written and illustrated by Osamu Tezuka and serialized 1973–1983.

4 Translators' note: References to fictional characters in various Japanese media. Zatōichi and Tange Sazen are mighty swordsmen referred to in multiple media forms: novels, TV dramas, films, performing arts, *manga*, etc. Zatōichi is blind, and Tange Sazen is one-eyed and one-armed. Captain Harlock (one-eyed) and Queen Emeraldas are cosmic pirates with scars on their faces.

5 Translators' note: Hōnen (1133–1212) was the founder of Japanese Pure Land Buddhism School called *Jōdo-shū*. He and his followers were all exiled by the emperor in 1207.

6 Translators' note: Known in English as the Great Hanshin or Kobe Earthquake. The earthquake, which registered a 6.9 on the moment magnitude scale, hit the southern portion of Hyōgo prefecture on Honshou Island in 1995.

7 Translators' note: *Henro* is both the Japanese word for "pilgrim" and the name of a famous pilgrimage route in Shikoku, Japan.

8 Translators' note: Important Japanese Buddhist monk who founded the True Word (*Shingon*) sect.

9 Translators' note: Morita Therapy is a form of psychotherapy developed by the Japanese psychiatrist Shōma Morita (1874–1938) as a treatment for neurotic anxiety. The goal of the therapy is to accept life as it is (*arugamama*).

Naikan Therapy (*naikan*: introspection) is a structured introspection process informed by Japanese Buddhism that was developed by Ishin Yoshimoto (1916–1988), a Buddhist monk of the Pure Land sect. It is designed to help individuals reflect on themselves and their relationships. The individual reflects on one relationship at a time by considering the following three questions: What have I received from this person? What have I given to this person? What troubles and difficulties have I caused this person?

10 Translators' note: The prominent leader who incited a revolution in the Bakumatsu Period (1853–1867). This occurred at the conclusion of the Edo Period (1603–1868), as the Tokugawa Shogunate was ending.

11 Translators' note: In the original Japanese, the image conjured up is that of passing a baton in a cosmic relay race, i.e., Christ passing on the work to Black Jack. Matsumoto (b. 1938) is a prolific Japanese author who developed

his own cosmology, which is referenced in this quote. The idea is that at a distant future time, future-time will meet up with past-time, thus forming a ring or loop.
12 Translators' note: A Japanese journalist and critic (b. 1939).
13 Translators' note: In addition to his training as a psychiatrist and Jungian analyst, the author is licensed as a clinical psychologist. Cf. endnote in Preface [English edition] regarding the discipline and licensure of clinical psychology in Japan.

References

Akita, I. (1997). Koseika-ni-okeru collectivity-to-individuality-shiron: "Tsumi"-to-koseika [The problem of collectivity and individuality on individuation: Guilt and individuation]. *Bulletin of the Kyoto Bunkyo Center for Clinical Psychology*, 23–30.

Akita, I. (2001). Shinriryōhō-to-ningen: Disfigured hero Shiron [Psychotherapy and human beings: A study on the disfigured hero]. In H. Kawai (Ed.), *Kōza shinriryōhō* [Psychotherapy course] (Vol. 6, pp. 111–153). Tokyo, Japan: Iwanami Shoten.

Matsumoto, L. (1990). *Galaxy Express 999* (Vol. 10). Tokyo, Japan: Shogakukan Sosho.

Moon, B. (Ed.) (1997). *An encyclopedia of archetypal symbolism: The archive for research in archetypal symbolism* (Vol. 1). Boston, MA: Shambhala Publications.

Morimoto, T. (1978). *Kotoba-eno-tabi* [Journey to words] (Vol. 3). Tokyo, Japan: Kadokawa Bunko.

Shiba, R. (1988). *Ryōma-ga-yuku* (Vol. 7). Tokyo, Japan: Bunshun Bunko. (Original work published 1962–1966)

Tezuka, O. (1987). Unexploded bomb (Episode 115). In *Black Jack* (Vol. 7, pp. 103–127). Tokyo, Japan: Akita shoten. (Original work published 1976)

Tezuka, O. (1988). The second person (Episode 195). In *Black Jack* (Vol. 12, pp. 133–153). Tokyo, Japan: Akita shoten. (Original work published 1977)

Yokoyama, T. (1988). Meikyū. In S. Kato (Ed.), *World Encyclopedia* (Vol. 28, pp. 12–13). Tokyo, Japan: Heibonsha.

Conclusion

From mental health to *psycheology*

Once people cross the first line, the resultant changes to body and mind may lead them to become personhood disordered. If the second line is crossed, they fall into a state that can be described as madness. People in this state are no longer "people" because even the quality of their souls has deteriorated. This is the real fear that arises when something like a personhood disorder infects the core of their being.

The state of a person who has crossed the second line is not necessarily the same as the state diagnosed with mental disorders. Sometimes one who has crossed the second line appears to be totally normal. The theory of clinical states, which sees pathology in phases from normal to neurotic to personhood disordered to psychotic, does not correspond to levels of madness. It does not correspond to the level of suffering, either. Psychotherapists become too dependent on this theory, while remaining ignorant regarding levels of madness and suffering. There are many therapists who are caught in the delusion that they have grasped everything about a given client. The theory of clinical states is useful as a perspective, but lacks the capacity to assess the level of madness and suffering by drawing upon the therapist's whole self.[1]

The mental health perspective remains rigidly fixed. The global expansion of this diagnostic system has only increased this tendency. The diagnostic perspective assesses people via symptoms. That method is not incorrect as a part of the mental health system. However, there are innumerable perspectives that can coexist with it.

Buddhism is one example. It is not right to abandon a perspective that has been preserved for 2,500 years. With its philosophy of karma and reincarnation, Buddhism has been substantiated through the understanding and appreciation of countless people. Is the Buddhist perspective inferior to that of mental health in terms of quality? No. Compared to the broad perspective and rich philosophy of Buddhism, the DSM and ICD are lamentably single-layered and superficial.

There is a troubling situation that can arise when this narrow mental health perspective carries decisive influence in judicial cases.

This occurs through the vehicle of mental health evaluations. It cannot be right to have the mental health perspective, which sees the world exclusively in terms of disease states, determine people's lives. When people are judged as insane or of diminished capacity, their charges are dropped or lessened in recognition of their inability to take responsibility for themselves. Insanity refers to the state in which an individual's ego cannot control the person. An example might be someone who committed murder while under the control of auditory hallucinations or delusions. In such a case, the person can avoid liability.

There are times, however, when the devil whispers to those who are not psychotic. Sometimes they yield to the whisper, kill someone, and are subsequently charged with the crime. The devil whispers in various ways. One way is to bring people to the state of psychosis first, then whisper. It is effective to whisper after weakening their ego. Yet, bringing them to the state of psychosis is not the only way to weaken the ego. Some cannot control their ego when a huge inheritance is dangled in front of them. Some cannot control themselves when the opportunity to acquire a high-ranking position is before them, or when they are heartbroken.

These are straightforward examples that are easy to understand. However, if we include the notion of one's fate from a previous incarnation, as in Buddhism, the situation becomes very complicated. What has influenced the person who committed the crime? The predicament leading up to the crime can be understood relatively easily. If the person's childhood home environment is taken into consideration, understanding the situation becomes a bit more complicated. If the person's former reincarnation is added to the mix, the situation transcends the framework of our current human understanding.

As far as Japanese people are concerned, no judgment should be made without some consideration of the Shinto and Buddhist perspectives, because these are foundational to their philosophy and existence. In this sense, the current approach to mental evaluation in Japan is undoubtedly wrong. The single-layered perspective of mental health was probably chosen unconsciously in an attempt to improve efficiency. It is a perfect solution for judging individuals who have committed sins and exacting justice smoothly.

We have much to learn from a situation in which a person, who was placed in extreme circumstances, took extreme action. It is in such situations that *psycheology*, which is essential to human beings, begins to take shape. Many such efforts can be found in the narrative world, including novels, *manga*, and cinema, but not in the judicial system of the real world. Images tend to precede reality. In sci-fi novels and *manga*, abundant images are provided first, and then reality follows.[2] The field of science also follows this process, where the tremendous enthusiasm and effort of scientists realize these images. Can we see such a drive in the field of justice? I have to say no, not enough. The field of justice must begin to follow the images, though belatedly. Those in the justice fields have a unique opportunity to understand the human experience through the extreme situations they encounter. Therefore, this knowledge will certainly contribute to the establishment of *psycheology*, which transcends the framework of mental health.

It is completely up to readers' judgment whether this book provides a "new wineskin" named *psycheology* or not. In making that judgment, however, it is worth bearing in mind that *psycheology* extends well beyond personhood disorders and psychopathy. Its perspective must be sufficiently broad to capture madness, lest it prove undeserving of its name.[3]

In concluding this book, I would like to present some ideas about possible future directions for my theory of madness. I would like to provide wandering madness with a place where it belongs, though this will involve some repetition and overlap with previous chapters.

I

What is madness?

At the root of this question's answer is human nature, which does not allow two heroes to stand on equal footing. "Two great heroes do not stand on an equal footing" or "Two heroes always fight against each other" ("Ryōyū [Two heroes]," 2012, pp. 1450–1451, our translation) are proverbs dating back to the *Records of the Grand Historian*, the *Tale of the Heike*, and the *Book of Han*.[4] This fundamental spirit of human beings can also be seen in the West, of course, as in "When Greek meets Greek, then comes the tug of war" (Simpson & Speake, 2008, p. 142).

As long as the spirit that is alive in the depths of human beings concerns two heroes not standing on equal footing, we will continue to be controlled by madness. Not allowing two heroes to stand on equal footing sets in motion psychological dynamics that strive to determine one and only one hero. Unending massacres and wars throughout recorded human history are hideous expressions of what it is to be controlled by this dynamic. A similar dynamic is activated in smaller-scale violence and murder.

Now who or what are the two heroes? In plain language, they represent the strong versus the strong, or the hero versus the hero; but how can this be said in depth psychological terms?

Depth psychology and its big brother, psychiatric medicine, were born and raised in the West. In their words, it would be something like conscious versus unconscious, ego versus shadow, or more generally, normal versus abnormal, health versus disease, symptomatic and asymptomatic, and so on. The idea of "two great heroes do not stand on an equal footing" can also be seen here. The conscious must conquer the unconscious. The ego (which controls consciousness) should not be defeated by the shadow (which is the negative side of human beings). Abnormalities, diseases, and symptoms must also be defeated.

Psycheology proposes the idea of "two heroes stand on equal footing" to protest against the dynamics of not letting two heroes stand on equal footing, which is a fundamental driver for both depth psychology and psychiatric medicine. The protest is important because the principle of "two heroes stand on equal footing" is the only one (i.e., compared to focusing on symptoms) that can guide human beings out of madness.

I stated my idea about human nature from the depth psychological perspective first, even though it might be harder to take in right away. Let's rise up to the level of common sense, which is easier, to consider the question and make a response once again.

II

What is madness?

It is a sense of strangeness felt by society.[5] Individuals belong to society. They cannot help belonging to a society, with very few exceptions.

As Kinya Abe (1995) has pointed out, the word "society" is better considered as "public spirit"[6] in the case of Japan. Public spirit, however, deeply includes individuality, so the antonym for "individual" is society rather than public spirit. In *No Longer Human*, for instance, one of the protagonists was blamed by his playmates: "The public spirit won't allow that," they said. "It is not the public spirit," said the protagonist, "but you who cannot allow that" (Dazai, 1948/1961, p. 408, our translation). And he began to think that the public spirit was actually individual. This is an example of the individuality in the public spirit.[7]

Society is a collective entity composed of individuals with a clear boundary. A society – a literary or medical society, The Society of Friends, The Society of Jesus, etc. – specifies its members and clearly delineates those who belong and those who do not.

What about public spirit, then? It is quite different from society. For some individuals, public spirit means family, friends, relatives, neighbors in the same village or town, etc., and its circle expands from there. For other individuals, like the protagonist in *No Longer Human*, public spirit means individuals themselves. Where public spirit begins and ends is difficult to define.

In this sense, society is still more befitting as the antonym of individual than public spirit. If the Japanese terms for individual (*kojin*) and society (*shakai*) are traced back to their origins, they were coined as translated words from Western languages. Therefore, it is understandable to consider the individual and society as antonyms.

As stated previously, madness is a sense of strangeness felt by society. Society at large, however, consciously and unconsciously delegated the description and interpretation of "a sense of strangeness" to the psychiatric society. This gave rise to the psychiatric diagnostic system.

Here comes another big problem, which is also global and universal.

A "sense of strangeness" can signify either one's first sensations or a deeper movement to exclude minorities. Majorities try to exclude this "sense of strangeness" almost unconsciously. In its depths, psychiatric symptomatology, which arose from these deep psychodynamics, is also controlled by the excluding attitude. Plus, the problems of society and public spirit are added here in Japan. One can see in ostracism the public spirit's immeasurable power to exclude in Japan. And it is difficult to determine the primary influences in this exclusion.

What about a "sense of strangeness felt in society by individuals" as a contrast to a "sense of strangeness felt by society"? It is easier to verbalize a sense of strangeness "in society" that is felt by individuals, since a society has regulations and rules. People can state their opinions candidly in response to such regulations and rules with relative ease.

However, what about a "sense of strangeness felt in the public spirit by individuals"? Expressing an objection to the public spirit is extremely difficult in Japan, so people have to sense how those around them (public spirit) think – not only sense, but behave according to this sense. Or they have to handle situations by catching a whiff of the majority opinion, which has been constructed behind closed doors.[8] Society has the power to oppress individuals, but in Japan individuals are oppressed by both society and the public spirit.

Madness is a sense of strangeness felt by society, but individuals also feel madness in society and the public spirit. It may create an oppressive feeling, and depending on the type and degree of this oppressive feeling, mental disorders or even madness may occur.

If you were asked who a professional in madness is, how would you answer?

Philosophers, psychologists, literary people, theologians, and legal scholars might all be potential candidates, yet the pool gradually settles into either mental health professionals or mental health researchers. This is because people involved with mental health are considered to be those who meet the mad most often.

This recognition, however, is wrong from the beginning. A mental health professional is an expert in mental disorders, not madness. More specifically, a mental health professional is not an expert in the nature of madness, but an expert who tries to help people considered to be suffering from mental disorders. And yet, there is no academic field specializing in madness;[9] so it probably fell to mental health professionals, onto whose profession of mental disorders people are liable to project madness. There is far too little social recognition of this fact. I emphasize this point because I want it to be well recognized.

Psychiatrists have been developing the diagnostic system they use for a very long time. It is the "operational diagnostic criteria" system, which is designed to allow anyone to reach the same diagnosis, that currently dominates the globe. The eye of these diagnostic criteria is not the eye of the public spirit (which is strongly colored by individuality) but the eye of society – more specifically, the psychiatric medicine society. This fact needs to be recognized as well.

III

Needless to say, madness – and thus human beings – cannot be measured on a universal scale. Nevertheless, the present global trend is obsessed with establishing a universal measure. This pursuit of universals for psychiatric diagnostic criteria began when psychiatric medicine became a part of the medical field. All of the medical branches, with the exception of psychiatric medicine, relate to the human body and deal with the physical. Psychiatric medicine does not. It deals with the world before or after the physical. It is a fundamental error to employ the same scale used by the medical branches concerned with the human body. This is also something of which we need to be well aware.

In summary, the professional in madness is thought to be the mental health professional. The diagnostic criteria that clinicians use are constructed based on criteria used for the physical body. Addressing situations before or after the physical requires a different perspective, one that contemporary mental health lacks. This is why *psycheology* is so necessary.

What defines madness differs greatly by region and era, as madness is strongly influenced by subjectivity. It is typically considered madness when an individual – or society, for that matter – wanders from the course set by others. In this sense, madness has a strong dependence on orientation, arising in the gap between how an individual and his or her encompassing society orient themselves. This point overlaps with the issue of "a sense of strangeness" mentioned previously.

IV

Madness was locked up in the system of mental health under the term mental disorders. Madness was supposed to be a path to the source of the human psyche, captivating in itself. Instead, it was buried under the numerous mental disorders assigned to describe it, locked up by the attention given to symptomatology in its place. Madness has been constrained and locked up in mental health for more than a hundred years, just like the imp in the bottle.

It has become really difficult for human beings to live with, as well as live through, madness. The human psyche has become more constrained.

Why did all these things happen?

Because the existential level of madness has been misunderstood.

What is the nature of this misunderstanding?

Let's take a look at God and Buddha. These beings exist for people who believe in them, and do not for people who do not. That is, their presence is dependent on religious devotion. What about ghosts, spirits, and specters? They also exist for people who believe and do not for people who do not. They most likely exist in the same manner as God, the devil, or Buddha, in terms of their dependence on believers' faith.

What about UFOs, or mysterious animals like the Loch Ness Monster and the Himalayan Yeti? These are truly strange. They never show up, yet suggestive evidence is presented time and again: vague objects resembling a UFO, something akin to a dinosaur in the Lock Ness, or footprints presumed to be like the Yeti's. Such phenomena, too, exist for people who believe and do not for those who do not. I do not mean to be impolite, but their presence may be dependent on one's fondness for extraordinary events.

I can then expect the following counterstatement: "What if they are discovered?" The unidentified mysterious objects and animals are at a different existential level than deities and specters, which will almost never be discovered. Therefore, they also need to be considered a bit differently from deities and specters. As soon as they are discovered, a change in the existential level would arise. Then, their role at that existential level would be completed. This termination would be brought about by the transformation of human consciousness. As I mentioned in the Introduction, both the existential level and the formative experience[10] can be said to change when the present consciousness supporting them changes. This change in existential level is not limited to unidentified objects and mysterious animals.

Anyway, the beings dependent on religious devotion, UFOs, and the Lock Ness Monster do not operate at an existential level that can be explained with our present understanding of things. A totally new conception is required. Similarly, madness operates at a level where its existence is fatefully dependent upon one's subjectivity.

Nevertheless, madness (termed mental disorders today) is organized into the same system as physical diseases. In the domain of the physical body dealt with by somatic medicine, gastric cancer is given its proper place within the framework of somatic disease. Mental disorders are treated as if they were similar, but they involve a different dimension that requires a different kind of system. If madness is handled as if it were like gastric cancer, it remains locked up in the wrong system. Because madness involves philosophy of mind, it appears completely different depending on one's vantage point. Madness cannot be viewed like a painting on display in a museum. The question of how to present it is a real challenge. Its proper appreciation requires the flexibility to view it from various standpoints, and even dimensions.

Madness exists at an existential level that does not allow objectivity to come closer.

In addition, madness has the nature of exposing itself at the moment when the word "madness" is uttered. As soon as the phrase "You are mad" is uttered, madness appears. Where? It descends upon either the one who utters it or the one it is meant to describe. Or else, it descends upon and locks up both. It is also the same when madness is implied under the guise of mental disorders.

Some may think that I perceive today's psychiatric diagnostic system as something like the *Malleus Maleficarum* (*The Hammer of Witches*), the book used to "diagnose" witches at the trials in medieval Europe. Yes and no. Yes, in that today's diagnostic system does unfortunately have a side like the witch trials. Sometimes clinicians lock a person up in giving a diagnosis, and sometimes psychiatrists prescribe an antipsychotic drug in order to restrain a person's psyche. No, in that clinicians do not burn clients at the stake in using diagnoses. Clinicians try to help clients, though they may be beyond their reach. On the other hand, it can also be said that helping professionals have put great effort into establishing the mental health system, which was finally successful in locking up madness. It is not safe to have madness fully released.

It is inappropriate to keep madness locked up, yet it is troublesome if madness is released.

What, then, should we do?

A place for madness

Finding a proper home for madness is our final topic. Madness has been displaced. There were times when madness temporarily resided in theology, as well as philosophy. After a great passage of time, it has been settling down, or has already settled, in mental health. However, this is not the proper place for madness. Where, then, should it reside? Madness should be in the arts. And it has already found some shelter there.

Take a look at *Kabuki*. Chillingly, there is an "aesthetic of killing" in the world of *Kabuki*. A *Kabuki* actor might enact the unmerciful slaughter of numerous people. In addition, the villain kills the hero, or the innocent. It is not the hero wiping out the villain, yet the audience gives a loud ovation to such a show and actor. This is because the madness of killing is sublimated into beauty, though it is chilling. The audience is completely absorbed in the actors' exquisite portrayal of mad killing, intoxicated by their flowers of evil.[11] This is where madness primarily belongs. The "beauty of madness"[12] exists in art.

This beauty of madness can be seen in the last scene of *The Love Suicides at Sonezaki*[13] (1703/2006), written by Chikamatsu Monzaemon, although it is not a story about killing others. In Ohatsu and Tokubei's scene, Ohatsu cries, "'Hurry up – kill me, kill me!' How beautiful the countenance of Ohatsu's determined mind" (p. 100, our translation). This play about the love suicides of Ohatsu and Tokubei depicts a mad situation with great beauty. It is also an example of the beauty of madness. People in the Edo period[14] gave frantic cheers to this scene of love suicides. No problem so far. However, the madness played out in reality: people were influenced and numerous love suicides took place. It is important to pay close attention here. The beauty of madness connected the theatrical scene to reality. Images and beauty have such power.

Mental health, where madness has been settling down, is reality. When its labels and concepts are applied, madness misunderstands them as roles to be performed. Thus, mental health and its labeling of mental disorders increase the possibility of madness getting released into reality. Most important of all, the names of mental diseases are not actors' professional names,[15] which would allow us to perform madness. Mental health does not prepare the stage for that. When the "madness archetype" in the depths mistakes the name of a disease as its role or its professional acting name, madness will feel miserably hurt, as no stage is prepared there.

Once again, I reiterate the point.

The place for madness is in the arts. There, numerous stages of a suitable nature can be found on which madness can play itself out. Madness should not extend out to reality, but dance fully and freely with various characters on the stage.[16] Finding expression in reality is not allowed except when madness is woven into the most noble of human endeavors.

Notes

1 Translators' note: i.e., making use of all available modes of information a therapist might access.

2 Translators' note: The argument is that imagination precedes reality. In other words, the creative arts provide images that seed the reality we subsequently create.
3 Translators' note: See endnote in Preface [Japanese edition] regarding meaning of *psycheology*.
4 Translators' note: The *Records of the Grand Historian* (*Shih-chi*) is the court historian Sima Qian's account of ancient Chinese history, written around 91 B.C.
The *Tale of the Heike* (*Taiheiki*) is a Japanese historical epic depicting the period 1319–1367 A.D. It was written in the late 14th century by an unknown author.
The *Book of Han* (*Han-shu*, known as the *Kanjo* in Japan) is a Chinese historical record of the Former (Western) Han Dynasty (206 B.C.–8 A.D.), edited during the Latter (Eastern) Han Dynasty (25–220 A.D.).
5 Translators' note: The *Random House Dictionary of the English Language* defines "society" as 1) "an organized group of persons associated together for religious, benevolent, cultural, scientific, political, patriotic, or other purposes," and 2) "a body of individuals living as members of a community" ("society," 1966).
In terms of the author's usage, *shakai* ("society") is consistent with the first definition of the term given above. In contrast, *seken* ("public spirit") is roughly equivalent to the second definition of "society."
6 Translators' note: *Seken* is a term distinctive to Japanese culture. Roughly translated, *seken* means "world around you." It has also been translated as "world," "society," "public," or "life." In this work, it is translated as "public spirit."
Seken originated as a Buddhist term for all the living things and elements surrounding us. In terms of daily experience, *seken* signifies a given individual's sphere of interpersonal concern. It varies from person to person, but would generally involve several concentric rings of social influence: from family, to the people with whom one often has contact, to the broader social sphere.
7 Translators' note: i.e., the individual would be just another, smaller concentric ring housed within family (cf. previous endnote).
8 Translators' note: In Japan, coming to a communal decision (whether in the personal or professional sphere) occurs primarily behind the scenes in a series of conversations that precede the (formal) meeting where these decisions are settled.
9 Author's note: Forensic psychiatry might be thought of as the specialized field for madness, but the role of forensic psychiatry is primarily to evaluate the mental capacity of the accused in a psychiatric evaluation, and not to research the essence of madness.
10 Translators' note: The Japanese term used here is *gen-fūkei*, whereas *gen-taiken* is used in the Introduction. *Gen*: original, archaic; *fūkei*: scenery; and *taiken*: experience. While there is a slight difference in meaning that creates a certain resonance between the terms, the meaning is sufficiently similar to invite the use of the same phrase in translation.
11 Translators' note: An intentional reference to Baudelaire's *Les Fleurs du Mal.*
12 Translators' note: *Kyō-bi*. *Kyō*: madness; *bi*: beauty. Thus, a certain beauty to be found in madness or woundedness. This same phrase was translated as "mad beauty" in the Introduction and represents a new coinage by the author.
13 Translators' note: A *Bunraku* puppetry play. Chikamatsu Monzaemon, 1653–1724.
14 Translators' note: 1603–1868.

15 Translators' note: In the Japanese performing arts, top performers inherit professional names, which are passed down through generations of artists.
16 Translators' note: The passage references the stage metaphorically, i.e., it is intended to include the creative arts generally.

References

Abe, K. (1995). *Seken-towa-nanika* [What is *seken*?]. Tokyo, Japan: Kodansha Gendai Shinsho.

Dazai, O. (1961). *Ningen-shikkaku* [No longer human]. In S. Ito, K. Kamei, M. Nakamura, K. Hirano, & K. Yamamoto (Eds.), *Nihon gendai bungaku zenshū* (Vol. 88, pp. 376–429). Tokyo, Japan: Kodansha. (Original work published 1948)

Monzaemon, C. (2006). Sonezaki-shinjū [The love suicides at Sonezaki]. In Planning Board of the Graduate School of Literature and Human Sciences, Osaka City University (Ed.), *Kamigata bunka koza Sonezaki shinjū* (pp. 49–100). Osaka, Japan: Izumi Shoin. (Original work published 1703)

Ryōyū [Two heroes] (2012). In K. Kitamura (Ed.), *Koji-zokushin: Kotowaza-daijiten* [Historical events and popular beliefs: A dictionary of proverbs] (2nd ed., pp. 1450–1451). Tokyo, Japan: Shogakukan.

Simpson, J. & Speake, J. (Eds.) (2008). *A dictionary of proverbs* (5th ed.). New York, NY: Oxford University Press.

Society. (1966). In *The Random House dictionary of the English language* (unabridged ed.). New York, NY: Random House.

Postscript

In this book, I first proposed the concept of *psycheology.* Then, I discussed the *cause of existence* and posed questions regarding madness by using the concepts of personhood disorders and psychopathy. I also explained that the nature of madness involved disordered personhood as a result of pursuing godhood.

You may think that I, as a clinician, should have presented clinical cases or my clients' dreams. I rarely brought these up, but used many stories instead. I would like to express my deepest gratitude for these stories. They have always been an intimate part of my clinical work, and my life itself.

I also mentioned the terror of being locked up, with a focus on existence and madness. As discussed, the Minotaur was not locked up in the labyrinth because he was a monster. Anyone becomes a Minotaur if he or she is kept locked up.

The human psyche is connected to everything. That is, the scope of *psycheology* is such that it requires the study of everything, which is obviously impossible to do alone. Conversely, the good news is that everything can contribute to *psycheology*. Therefore, I plan to establish my own *psycheology* by studying what has been important to me, since providing a full foundation for it is beyond my reach. Nothing would make me happier than if my modest attempt contributed to those in the helping professions, as well as to those striving to live authentically.

It is too late to mention, but I used a term "personhood disorder" in this book. Personhood disorder (*jinkaku-shōgai*) was already in use as a mental health term when I first became a psychiatrist in 1985, which continued up until a few years ago when the term was officially replaced by "personality disorder" (personality-*shōgai*). Many mental health terms (including psychopathy, moral insanity, and degeneration theory) disappeared after being used for several decades. Personhood disorder has yet to die out completely, but it is disappearing. I ventured to use this term here because, in my several decades of clinical experience, I have met a number of clients whose suffering was aptly depicted by this term. I hope this book will be of some help to those whose suffering was, or still is, in keeping with disordered personhood.

Index

For Product Safety Concerns and Information please contact our EU representative GPSR@taylorandfrancis.com Taylor & Francis Verlag GmbH, Kaufingerstraße 24, 80331 München, Germany

Batch number: 10725973

Printed by Printforce, the Netherlands